Practical Manual of
Histology

As per Medical Council of India: Competency Based Undergraduate
Curriculum for the Indian Medical Graduate, 2018

Name ....
Year .... Roll no. ....
Name of the College ....
Teacher's Signature ....

This is to certify that Mr/Miss _____ 1st year MBBS student of batch _____
Has attained the knowledge and skill to identify all types of epithelia under the microscope and describe the various types that correlate to its function.

_____
Signature and seal of the Head
Department of Anatomy

_____
Signature and seal of the Dean

This is to certify that Mr/Miss _____ 1st year MBBS student of batch _____
Has attained the knowledge and skill to identify, draw and label a slide of trachea and lung.

_____
Signature and seal of the Head
Department of Anatomy

_____
Signature and seal of the Dean

Practical Manual of
Histology

As per Medical Council of India: Competency Based Undergraduate
Curriculum for the Indian Medical Graduate, 2018

Hina Sharma MBBS, MD (Anatomy)

Assistant Professor
Department of Anatomy
Geetanjali Medical College and Hospital
Udaipur, Rajasthan, India

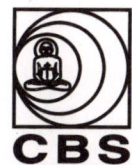

CBS

CBS Publishers & Distributors Pvt Ltd

New Delhi • Bengaluru • Chennai • Kochi • Kolkata • Mumbai
Bhopal • Bhubaneswar • Hyderabad • Jharkhand • Nagpur • Patna • Pune • Uttarakhand
Dhaka (Bangladesh) • Kathmandu (Nepal)

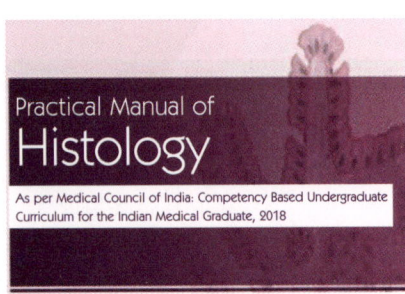

ISBN: 978-93-89396-61-4

First Edition: 2020

Published by Satish Kumar Jain and produced by Varun Jain for

CBS Publishers & Distributors Pvt Ltd

4819/XI Prahlad Street, 24 Ansari Road, Daryaganj, New Delhi 110 002, India.
Ph: 23289259, 23266861, 23266867 Website: www.cbspd.com
Fax: 011-23243014   e-mail: delhi@cbspd.com; cbspubs@airtelmail.in.

Corporate Office: 204 FIE, Industrial Area, Patparganj, Delhi 110 092

Ph: 011-4934 4934   Fax: 011-4934 4935   e-mail: publishing@cbspd.com; publicity@cbspd.com

Branches

- **Bengaluru:** Seema House 2975, 17th Cross, K.R. Road, Banasankari 2nd Stage, Bengaluru 560 070, Karnataka
  Ph: +91-80-26771678/79   Fax: +91-80-26771680   e-mail: bangalore@cbspd.com
- **Chennai:** 7, Subbaraya Street, Shenoy Nagar, Chennai 600 030, Tamil Nadu
  Ph: +91-44-26680620/26681266   Fax: +91-44-42032115   e-mail: chennai@cbspd.com
- **Kochi:** 42/1325, 1326, Power House Road, Opp KSEB, Power House, Ernakulam 682 018, Kochi, Kerala
  Ph: +91-484-4059061-65   Fax: +91-484-4059065   e-mail: kochi@cbspd.com
- **Kolkata:** 6/B, Ground Floor, Rameswar Shaw Road, Kolkata 700 014, West Bengal
  Ph: +91-33-22891126, 22891127, 22891128   e-mail: kolkata@cbspd.com
- **Mumbai:** 83-C, Dr E Moses Road, Worli, Mumbai 400018, Maharashtra
  Ph: +91-22-24902340/41   Fax: +91-22-24902342   e-mail: mumbai@cbspd.com

Representatives

• Bhopal	0-8319310552	• Bhubaneswar	0-9911037372	• Hyderabad	0-9885175004	• Jharkhand	0-9811541605
• Nagpur	0-9421945513	• Patna	0-9334159340	• Pune	0-9623451994	• Uttarakhand	0-9716462459
• Dhaka (Bangladesh)	01912-003485	• Kathmandu (Nepal)	977-9818742655				

Printed at: India Binding House, Greater Noida, UP India

Foreword

It gives me immense pleasure to introduce the *Practical Manual of Histology* as per the latest MCI syllabus. The author of this workbook has written it with the purpose of dealing with the practical aspects of identifying and describing the normal microanatomy of human tissues.

It has a good consortium of specific learning objectives, think and answer, three points of identification and hand-drawn diagrams. The author has addressed the problems encountered by the learners and penned this workbook in a way which will engender faster understanding of the subject.

I hope the students will take full advantage of the crisp dose of knowledge and diagrams provided in this workbook. At a first glance it looks very promising indeed and I wish the author success in her intent of making teaching and learning of histology a fruitful and rewarding experience.

Prof **FS Mehta** MS (General surgery)
Dean, Geetanjali Medical College and Hospital
Udaipur, Rajasthan
former Superintendent
Rabindra Nath Tagore Medical College and Hospital
Udaipur, Rajasthan, India

During the years of teaching histology I have experienced the difficulties encountered by the learners. There is a vast choice of literature for the students to pick from. The normal tendency to pick the easiest available means leads to notes borrowed from seniors. It leads to the problem seen in the whispering game—the end product is far from correct.

Another practical problem encountered is that the various textbooks offer various stains whereas the stain usually used and taught is haematoxylin and eosin (H & E). As such the learner is faced with the dilemma of which diagram to draw.

To address these issues the idea of promoting easy learning by providing hand-drawn diagrams of tissues stained with H & E stain was conceived. The diagrams are self-explanatory and help the learner identify the given tissue.

The highlight of this workbook is that it addresses all the latest competencies of histology given in the new curriculum.

Each slide has been given specific learning objectives. So at the very outset the learner knows what all he has to specifically look for in the given slide.

There are think and answer questions given at places to encourage the learner to use his/her grey cells because the mind sees what the brain knows. So once the learner begins with thinking he knows what to look for.

There is space provided for writing three points of identification of the slide. These will prove invaluable for last moment revision prior to assessments.

SDL pages have been provided for notes or diagrams. Sufficient space has been given to draw the diagrams with exemplary diagram above on the same page, thus removing the tedious process of turning pages to copy while drawing. If smaller diagram is to be drawn then a smaller circle may be drawn within the larger one.

This workbook is ideal for learning histology in various streams related to health education and is sufficient for preparation of viva voce.

Hina Sharma

Acknowledgements

Writing a book is by far harder than I first thought. None the less it is very rewarding. I thank the Almighty for giving me the opportunity to write this book.

I am eternally grateful to the management of Geetanjali Medical College for encouraging academic excellence and supporting in adopting newer methods of teaching. I specially am grateful to the Dean, Prof FS Mehta for initiating the idea of writing a workbook, without which I would probably have not even thought of it. He has been very supportive and inspired me to start this work.

Very special thanks to Prof Manjinder Kaur, Head, Department of Physiology, Geetanjali Medical College, for giving me the much required momentum to start writing this workbook. Being the academic officer, she has always been a source of stimulation for academic perfection.

I cannot thank my family enough for bearing with me and not being impatient when I could not do some of the chores due to preoccupation. Their constant support was the only reason that this workbook could be completed on time.

I am extremely grateful to Prof J Kain, Head, Department of Anatomy, for being supportive throughout this project.

My teacher and guide Prof LK Jain has always been a source of inspiration. The knowledge imparted by him is sound, complete and dependable. I thank him for his blessings.

My colleagues Dr Brijesh, Dr Charu, Dr Meghna and Dr Pritesh have provided an amicable environment and encouraged and appreciated my work. I am very grateful for their reinforcement.

My initial teaching years were very enriching and I thank my then colleagues Prof Ghanshyam Gupta, Prof Seema Prakash, Dr Parveen Ojha and Dr Pooja Dhabai for providing an academically inspiring environment.

I thank Prof GC Agarwal for helping me enhance my knowledge of histology during initial teaching years. He encouraged me to avoid taking a casual approach towards teaching histology.

I wholeheartedly thank Mrs Jyotsana, Mr Biju, Mr Bhagwati, Mr Vinod and Mr Jagdish for their support.

The students have always been a source of inspiration. I thank them for putting their faith in me and giving me the much required compliments.

I am grateful to all my friends for encouraging me to complete this workbook.

I thank the publisher, and the others involved for printing this workbook in such a short notice.

Hina Sharma

Contents

No.	Practical	Page no.	Teacher's signature	Remarks
	Endocrine Glands	275		
92	Pituitary Gland	275		
93	Thyroid Gland	278		
94	Parathyroid Gland	280		
95	Pineal Gland	283		
96	Suprarenal Gland	285		
	Central Nervous System	290		
97	Spinal Cord	290		
98	Cerebrum	293		
99	Cerebellum	295		
	Special Senses	299		
100	Cornea	300		
101	Sclero-corneal Junction	302		
102	Retina	305		
103	Optic Nerve	309		
104	Eyelid	311		
105	Lip	315		
106	Cochlea and Organ of Corti	317		

SUGGESTED ASSESSMENT CRITERIA

- Complete file with good and accurate diagrams — 5 marks
- Complete file but few (less than 10%) incorrect diagrams — 4 marks
- Complete file but mostly (more than 50%) incorrect diagrams — 3 marks
- Incomplete file (more than 75% complete) — 2 marks
- Incomplete file (less than 75% complete) — 1 mark
- No diagrams drawn (less than 25% diagrams drawn) — Zero

INDEX OF COMPETENCIES FOR HISTOLOGY

Note: Competency numbers are as provided in the new curriculum.

LIGHT MICROSCOPE

LABEL THE PARTS OF THE MICROSCOPE

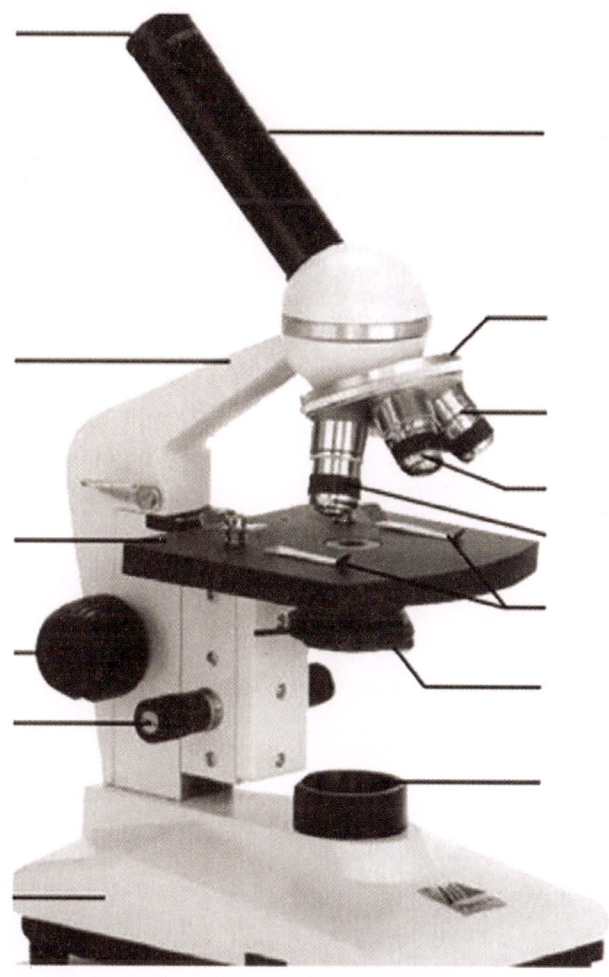

SPECIFIC LEARNING OBJECTIVES

At the end of the session the student should be able to:
1. Identify all parts of the microscope.
2. Tell the functions of all the parts.
3. Attain the skill to focus a given slide at low and high power.

ACTIVITY

1. Focus the given slide in low power (10X)
2. Focus the given slide in high power (40X)

Viva Questions

1. Name the various types of microscopes

_____

_____

_____

_____

2. Name the parts of a light microscope used in your lab.

_____

_____

_____

_____

3. What are the magnifications available in the given light microscope? Which ones are commonly used?

_____

_____

_____

_____

4. How do you focus a slide on a light microscope?

_____

_____

_____

_____

5. What precautions are taken while focussing a slide in the light microscope?

_____

_____

_____

_____

_____

Date:

6. Which magnification is used first while focussing a slide?

_____

_____

_____

_____

SHOW HOW

1. Show how you adjust the lens for coarse focussing.
2. Show how you adjust the lens for fine focussing.
3. Which side of the slide do you keep upwards?

Note

Whenever you focus and try to identify a slide, always see the whole tissue by moving the slide on the stage of the microscope. Do not comment on the slide by looking at just one field.

Date:

EPITHELIUM HISTOLOGY

Number	Competency	Domain	Level	Core (Y/N)	Teaching/ learning method	Assessment method	Number required to certify
AN 65.1	Identify epithelium under the microscope and describe the various types that correlate to its function	K/S	P	Y	Lecture, practical	Written/skill assessment	1

SPECIFIC LEARNING OBJECTIVES

At the end of the session the student should be able to:

1. Classify different types of epithelia.

CLASSIFICATION OF EPITHELIUM

Answer the Following

Simple Epithelium (Single Layer of Cells)

Flat cells (squamous)

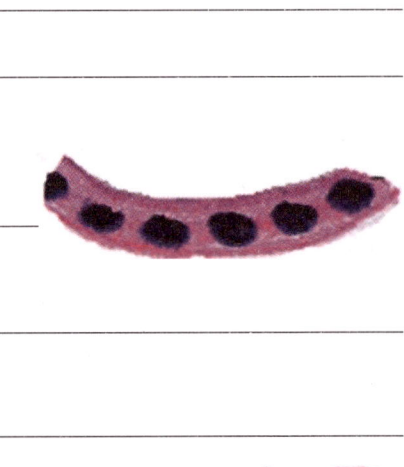

1. For example _____

2. What is the shape of the nucleus in such cells?

   _____

3. What is endothelium?_____

4. What is mesothelium?_____

Cells with equal height and width (cuboidal)

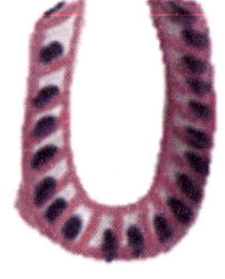

5. For example _____

6. What is the shape of the nucleus in such cells?

   _____

7. Where does the basement membrane lie?

   _____

Cells with height more than width (columnar)

8. For example _____

9. What is the shape of the nucleus in such cells?

   _____

10. Where does the basement membrane lie?

    _____

Stratified Epithelium (Multilayered Cells)

Stratified squamous epithelium

11. Shape of deeper layer of cells is:

_____

12. What is the shape of the nucleus in such cells?

_____

13. Shape of surface layer of cells is:

_____

14. For example

_____

15. Where does the basement membrane lie?

_____

Stratified cuboidal epithelium

16. Shape of deeper layer of cells is:

_____

17. What is the shape of the nucleus in such cells?

_____

18. Shape of surface layer of cells is:

_____

19. For example

_____

20. Where does the basement membrane lie?

_____

Stratified columnar epithelium

21. Shape of deeper layer of cells is:

_____

22. What is the shape of the nucleus in such cells?

_____

23. Shape of surface layer of cells is:

_____

24. For example

_____

25. Where does the basement membrane lie?

_____

Date:

Transitional epithelium

26. Shape of deeper layer of cells is:

_____

27. What is the shape of the nucleus in such cells?

_____

28. Shape of surface layer of cells is:

_____

29. What is the shape and number of nuclei in such cells?

_____

30. Where does the basement membrane lie?

_____

31. What is urothelium?

_____

_____

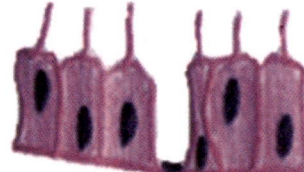

Pseudostratified epithelium

32. How many layers of cells are there in such epithelium?

_____

33. Why is it known as pseudostratified?

_____

Date:

SIMPLE SQUAMOUS EPITHELIUM

SPECIFIC LEARNING OBJECTIVES

At the end of the session the student should be able to:
1. Describe the characteristic features of simple epithelium.
2. Describe the shape of cells and nuclei in simple squamous epithelium.
3. Identify simple squamous epithelium under light microscope.
4. Give examples of tissues with squamous epithelium.
5. Describe the function of simple squamous epithelium and how the shape helps in doing so.
6. Draw a diagram showing microanatomy of simple squamous epithelium.

Distribution and function

_____

_____

_____

_____

Three points of identification

_____

_____

_____

_____

_____

_____

Date:

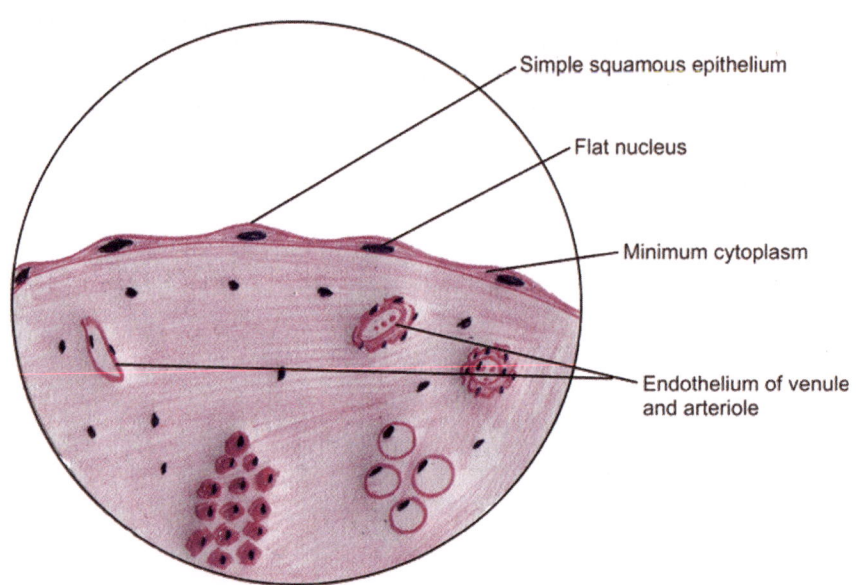

Simple squamous epithelium

Flat nucleus

Minimum cytoplasm

Endothelium of venule
and arteriole

Date:

SIMPLE CUBOIDAL EPITHELIUM

SPECIFIC LEARNING OBJECTIVES

At the end of the session the student should be able to:

1. Describe the shape of cells and nuclei in simple cuboidal epithelium.
2. Identify simple cuboidal epithelium under light microscope.
3. Give examples of tissues with cuboidal epithelium.
4. Draw a diagram showing microanatomy of simple cuboidal epithelium.

Distribution and function

_____

_____

_____

_____

Three points of identification

_____

_____

_____

_____

_____

_____

Date:

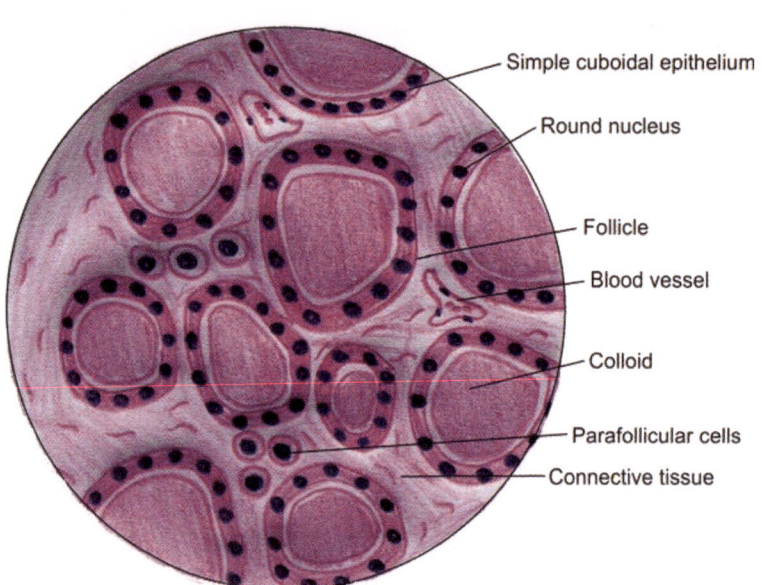

Simple cuboidal epithelium

Round nucleus

Follicle

Blood vessel

Colloid

Parafollicular cells

Connective tissue

Date:

SIMPLE COLUMNAR EPITHELIUM

SPECIFIC LEARNING OBJECTIVES

At the end of the session the student should be able to:

1. Describe the shape of cells and nuclei in simple columnar epithelium.
2. Identify simple columnar epithelium under light microscope.
3. Give examples of tissues with columnar epithelium.
4. Draw a diagram showing microanatomy of simple columnar epithelium.

Distribution and function

_____

_____

_____

_____

Three points of identification

_____

_____

_____

_____

_____

_____

Date:

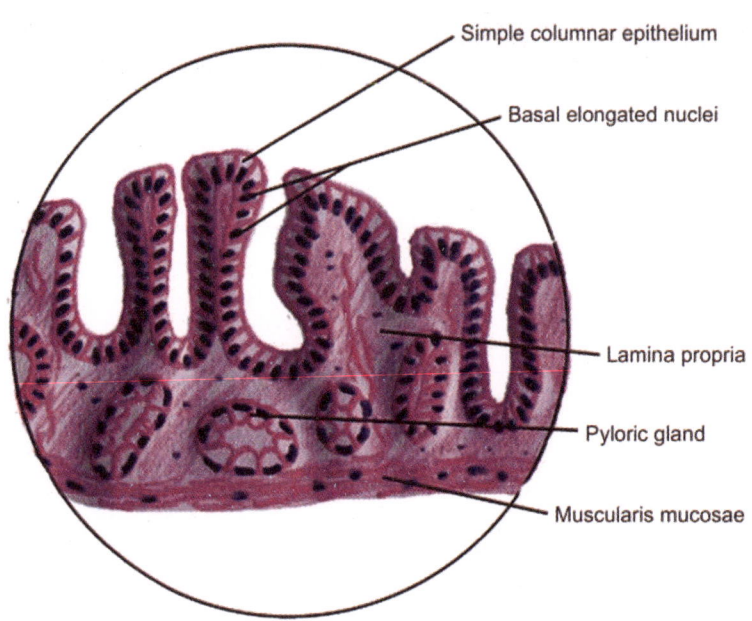

Simple columnar epithelium

Basal elongated nuclei

Lamina propria

Pyloric gland

Muscularis mucosae

Date:

SIMPLE CILIATED COLUMNAR EPITHELIUM

SPECIFIC LEARNING OBJECTIVES

At the end of the session the student should be able to:

1. Describe the shape of cells and nuclei in simple ciliated columnar epithelium.
2. Identify simple ciliated columnar epithelium under light microscope.
3. Give examples of tissues with ciliated columnar epithelium.
4. Describe the function of simple ciliated columnar epithelium.
5. Draw a diagram showing microanatomy of simple ciliated columnar epithelium.

Distribution and function

_____

_____

_____

_____

Three points of identification

_____

_____

_____

_____

_____

_____

Date:

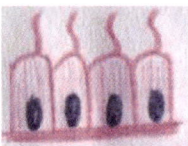

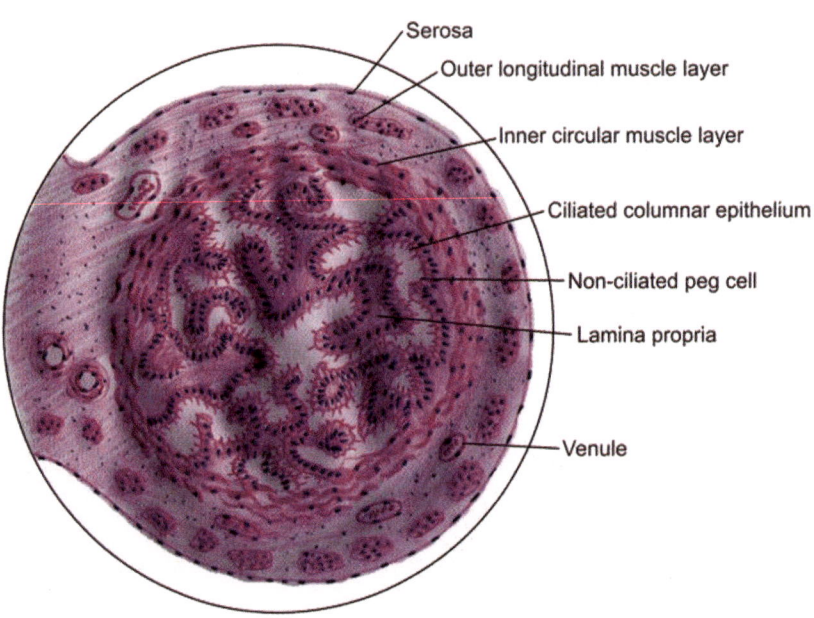

- Serosa
- Outer longitudinal muscle layer
- Inner circular muscle layer
- Ciliated columnar epithelium
- Non-ciliated peg cell
- Lamina propria
- Venule

Date:

SIMPLE COLUMNAR EPITHELIUM WITH BRUSH/STRIATED BORDER

SPECIFIC LEARNING OBJECTIVES

At the end of the session the student should be able to:

1. Describe the appearance of brush/striated border under light microscope.
2. Identify simple columnar epithelium with brush/striated border under light microscope.
3. Give examples of tissues with columnar epithelium with brush/striated border.
4. Describe the function of simple columnar epithelium with brush border.
5. Differentiate between brush border and striated border.
6. Explain what microvilli are.
7. Draw a diagram showing microanatomy of simple columnar epithelium with brush/striated border.

Distribution and function

_____

_____

_____

_____

Three points of identification

_____

_____

_____

_____

_____

_____

Date:

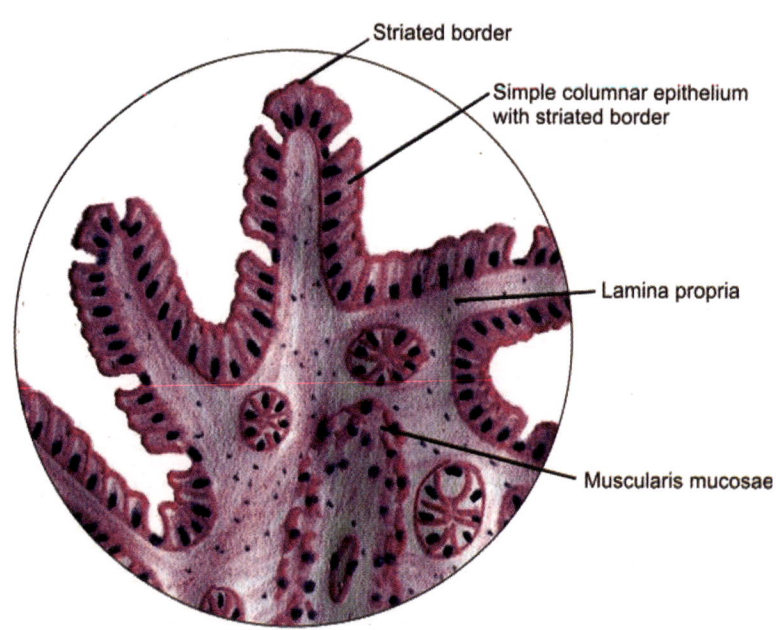

Striated border

Simple columnar epithelium
with striated border

Lamina propria

Muscularis mucosae

Date:

SDL NOTES

Date:

SDL NOTES

Date:

STRATIFIED SQUAMOUS EPITHELIUM (NON KERATINIZED)

SPECIFIC LEARNING OBJECTIVES

At the end of the session the student should be able to:

1. Describe the shape of cells and nuclei in stratified squamous epithelium.
2. Identify stratified squamous epithelium (non-keratinized) under light microscope.
3. Give examples of tissues with stratified squamous epithelium.
4. Describe the function of stratified squamous epithelium.
5. Draw a diagram showing microanatomy of stratified squamous epithelium (non-keratinized).

Distribution and function

_____

_____

_____

_____

Three points of identification

_____

_____

_____

_____

_____

_____

Date:

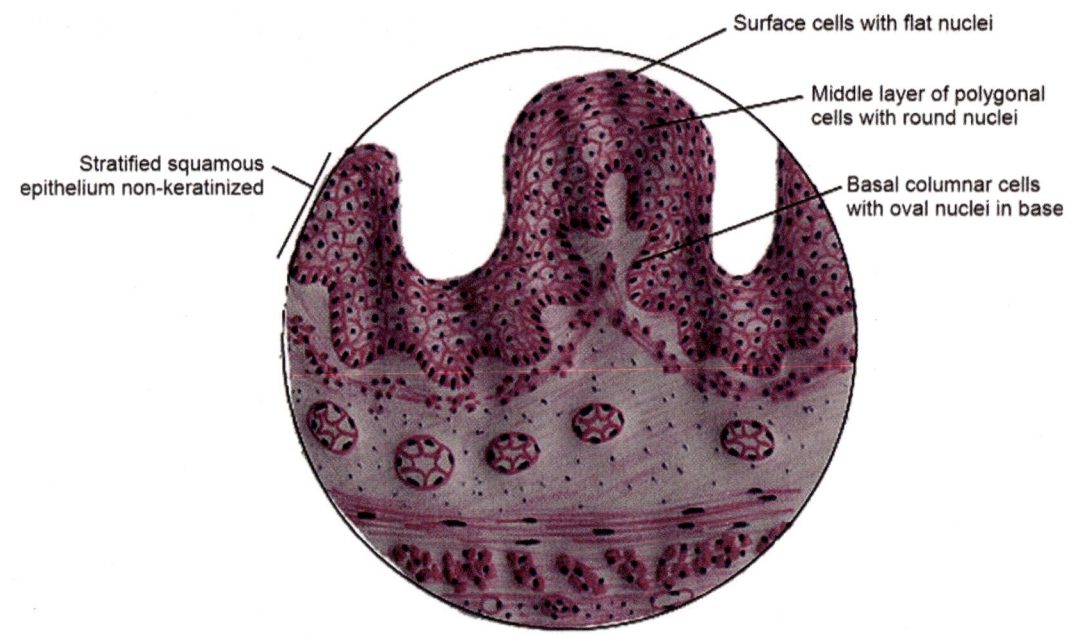

Surface cells with flat nuclei

Middle layer of polygonal cells with round nuclei

Stratified squamous epithelium non-keratinized

Basal columnar cells with oval nuclei in base

Date:

STRATIFIED SQUAMOUS EPITHELIUM (KERATINIZED)

SPECIFIC LEARNING OBJECTIVES

At the end of the session the student should be able to:

1. Describe the shape of cells and nuclei in stratified squamous keratinized epithelium.
2. Identify stratified squamous epithelium (keratinized) under light microscope.
3. Give examples of tissues with stratified squamous keratinized epithelium.
4. Describe the function of stratified squamous epithelium.
5. Draw a diagram showing microanatomy of stratified squamous epithelium (keratinized).

Distribution and function

_____

_____

_____

_____

Three points of identification

_____

_____

_____

_____

_____

_____

Date:

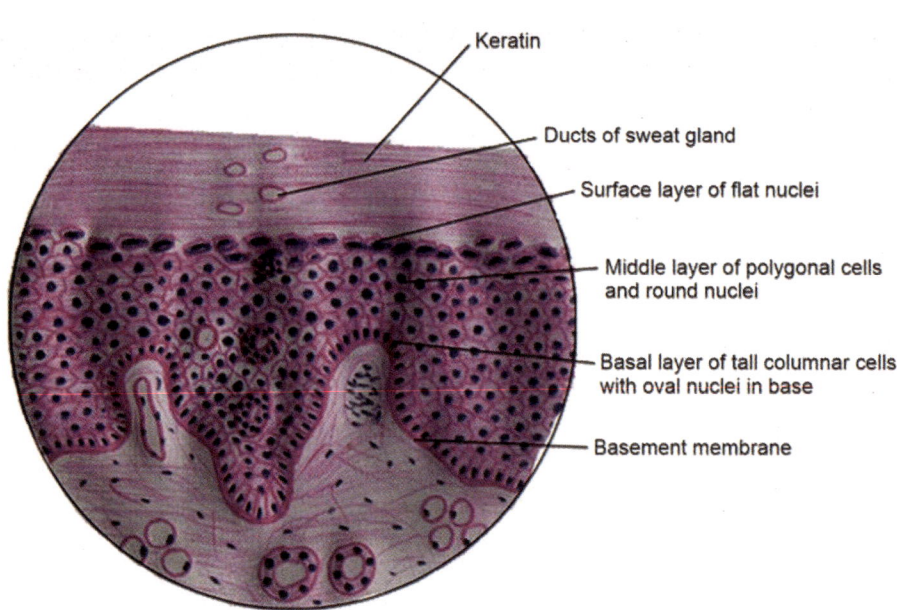

- Keratin
- Ducts of sweat gland
- Surface layer of flat nuclei
- Middle layer of polygonal cells and round nuclei
- Basal layer of tall columnar cells with oval nuclei in base
- Basement membrane

Date:

STRATIFIED CUBOIDAL EPITHELIUM

SPECIFIC LEARNING OBJECTIVES

At the end of the session the student should be able to:

1. Describe the shape of cells and nuclei in stratified cuboidal epithelium.
2. Identify stratified cuboidal epithelium under light microscope.
3. Give examples of tissues with stratified cuboidal epithelium.
4. Describe the function of stratified cuboidal epithelium.
5. Draw a diagram showing microanatomy of stratified cuboidal epithelium.

Distribution and function

_____

_____

_____

_____

Three points of identification

_____

_____

_____

_____

_____

_____

Date:

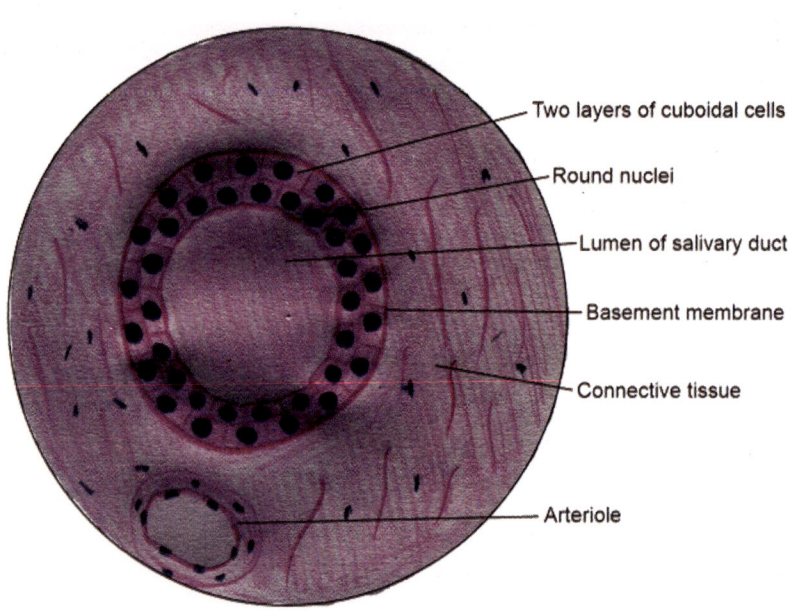

- Two layers of cuboidal cells
- Round nuclei
- Lumen of salivary duct
- Basement membrane
- Connective tissue
- Arteriole

Date:

STRATIFIED COLUMNAR EPITHELIUM

SPECIFIC LEARNING OBJECTIVES

At the end of the session the student should be able to:

1. Describe the shape of cells and nuclei in stratified columnar epithelium.
2. Identify stratified columnar epithelium under light microscope.
3. Give examples of tissues with stratified columnar epithelium.
4. Describe the function of stratified columnar epithelium.
5. Draw a diagram showing microanatomy of simple columnar epithelium.

Distribution and function

_____

_____

_____

_____

Three points of identification

_____

_____

_____

_____

_____

_____

Date:

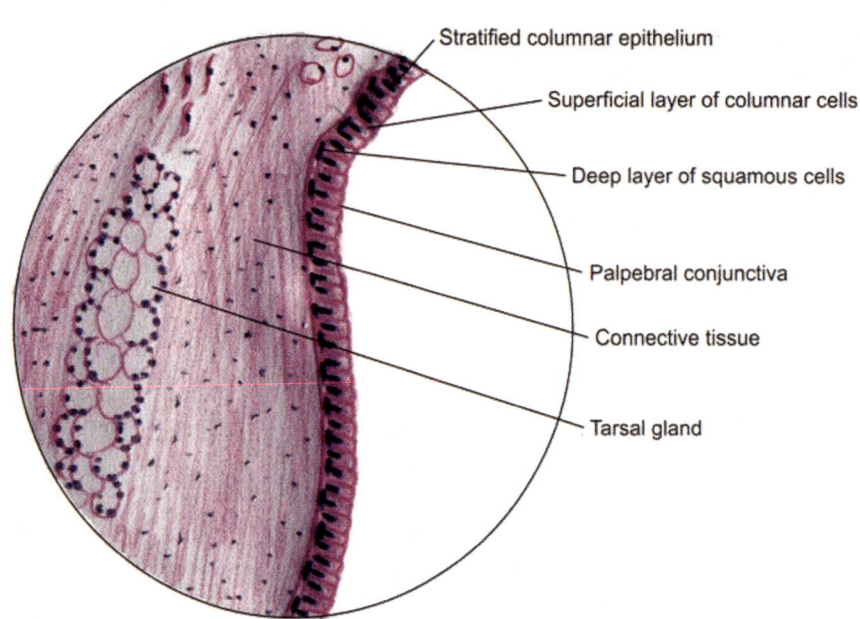

Stratified columnar epithelium

Superficial layer of columnar cells

Deep layer of squamous cells

Palpebral conjunctiva

Connective tissue

Tarsal gland

Date:

SDL NOTES

Date:

SDL NOTES

Date:

TRANSITIONAL EPITHELIUM (UNSTRETCHED BLADDER)

SPECIFIC LEARNING OBJECTIVES

At the end of the session the student should be able to:

1. Describe the shape of cells and nuclei in transitional epithelium in a contracted/unstretched bladder.
2. Identify transitional epithelium under light microscope.
3. Give examples of tissues with transitional epithelium.
4. Describe the function of transitional epithelium.
5. Tell if there is a basement membrane in urothelium.
6. Draw a diagram showing microanatomy of transitional epithelium of unstretched bladder.

Distribution and function

_____

_____

_____

_____

Three points of identification

_____

_____

_____

_____

_____

_____

Date:

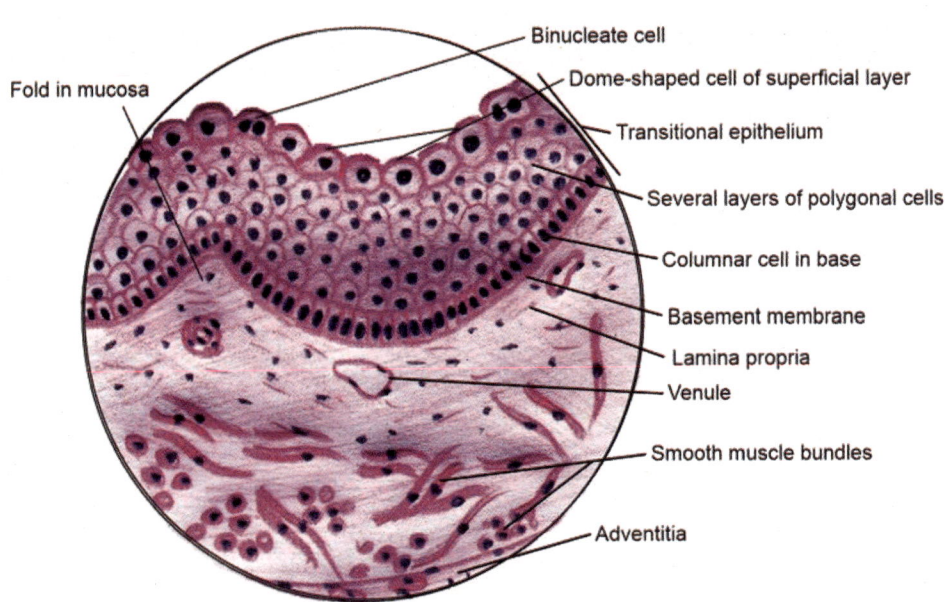

Fold in mucosa

Binucleate cell

Dome-shaped cell of superficial layer

Transitional epithelium

Several layers of polygonal cells

Columnar cell in base

Basement membrane

Lamina propria

Venule

Smooth muscle bundles

Adventitia

Date:

TRANSITIONAL EPITHELIUM (STRETCHED BLADDER)

SPECIFIC LEARNING OBJECTIVES

At the end of the session the student should be able to:

1. Describe the shape of cells and nuclei in transitional epithelium in a stretched bladder.
2. Identify transitional epithelium under light microscope.
3. Draw a diagram showing microanatomy of transitional epithelium of stretched bladder.

Three points of identification

_____

_____

_____

_____

_____

_____

Date:

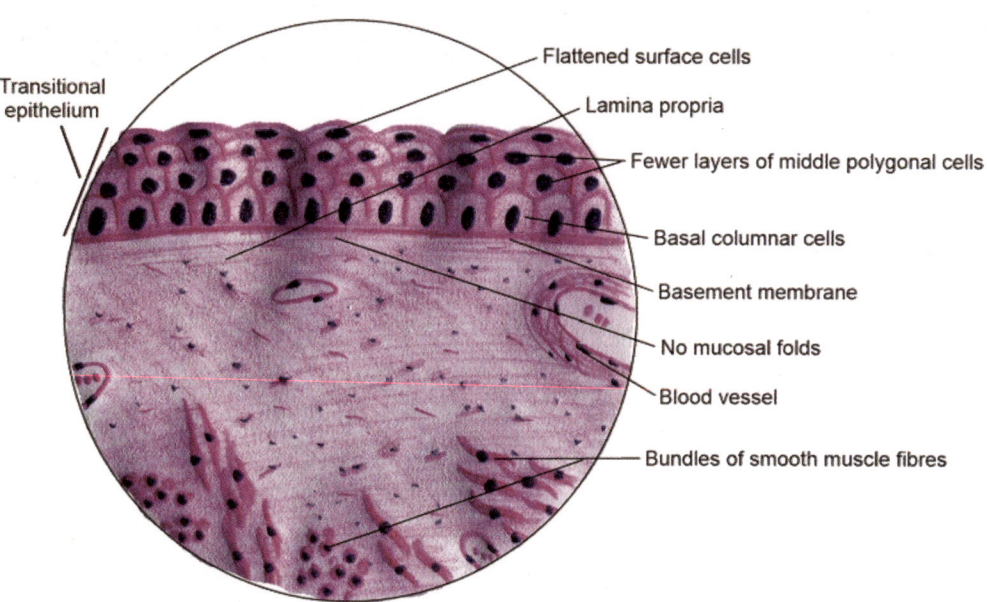

Transitional
epithelium

Flattened surface cells

Lamina propria

Fewer layers of middle polygonal cells

Basal columnar cells

Basement membrane

No mucosal folds

Blood vessel

Bundles of smooth muscle fibres

Date:

PSEUDOSTRATIFIED CILIATED COLUMNAR EPITHELIUM

SPECIFIC LEARNING OBJECTIVES

At the end of the session the student should be able to:

1. Describe the shape of cells and nuclei in pseudostratified columnar epithelium.
2. Give examples of tissues with pseudostratified ciliated columnar epithelium.
3. Describe what cilia are.
4. Describe the function of this epithelium.
5. Draw a diagram showing microanatomy of pseudostratified ciliated columnar epithelium.

Distribution and function

_____

_____

_____

_____

Three points of identification

_____

_____

_____

_____

_____

_____

Date:

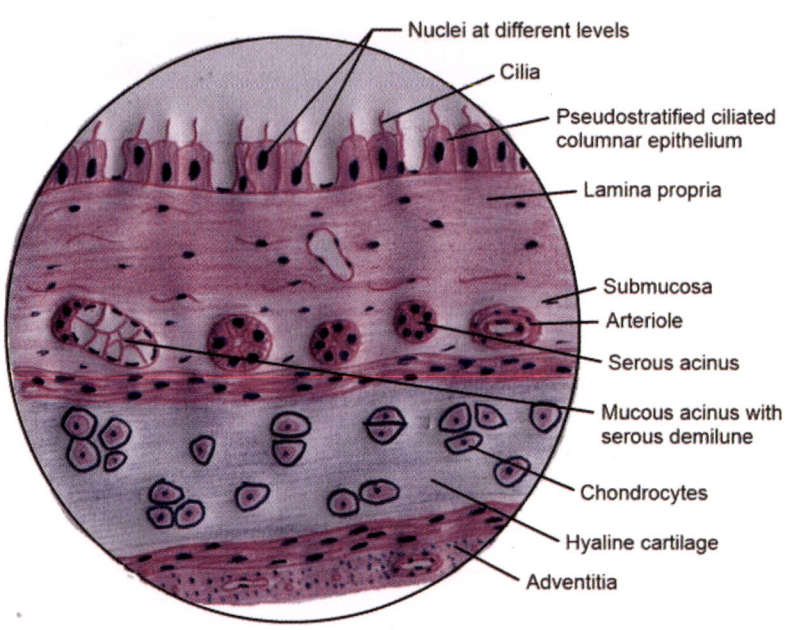

Nuclei at different levels

Cilia

Pseudostratified ciliated columnar epithelium

Lamina propria

Submucosa

Arteriole

Serous acinus

Mucous acinus with serous demilune

Chondrocytes

Hyaline cartilage

Adventitia

Date:

OLFACTORY EPITHELIUM

Number	Competency	Domain	Level	Core (Y/N)	Teaching/learning method	Assessment method	Number required to certify
AN 43.2	Identify, describe and draw the microanatomy of pituitary gland, thyroid, parathyroid gland, tongue, salivary glands, tonsil, epiglottis, cornea, retina	K/S	SH	Y	Lecture, practical	Written/skill assessment	

- Olfactory epithelium is present on the superior nasal concha and adjacent nasal septum near the roof of nasal cavity.
- The epithelium is pseudostratified. The superficial cytoplasm appears clear and the nuclear layer shows many rows of nuclei.
- Nuclei of olfactory cells are round. The superficial parts of these cells have non-motile olfactory cilia.
- Other cells of epithelium are sustentacular cells and basal cells.
- Lamina propria lies deep to epithelium. It has blood capillaries, lymphatics, nerves, and serous glands called Bowman's glands.

Date:

SPECIFIC LEARNING OBJECTIVES

At the end of the session the student should be able to:

1. Identify olfactory epithelium under the light microscope.
2. Identify pseudostratified epithelium of olfactory mucosa.
3. Identify olfactory neuron.
4. Identify sustentacular and basal cells.
5. Identify Bowman's glands.
6. Draw a diagram of microanatomy of olfactory epithelium.

Distribution and function

_____

_____

_____

_____

Three points of identification

_____

_____

_____

_____

_____

_____

Date:

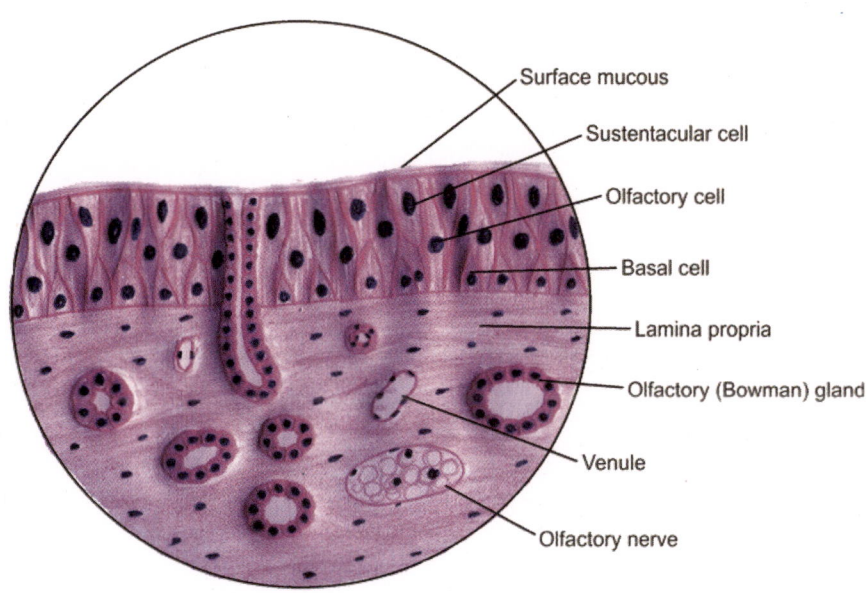

Surface mucous

Sustentacular cell

Olfactory cell

Basal cell

Lamina propria

Olfactory (Bowman) gland

Venule

Olfactory nerve

Date:

SDL NOTES

Date:

SDL NOTES

Date:

ULTRASTRUCTURE OF EPITHELIUM

Number	Competency	Domain	Level	Core (Y/N)	Teaching/learning method	Assessment method	Number required to certify
AN 65.2	Describe the ultrastructure of epithelium	K	KH	N	Lecture, practical	Written	

SPECIFIC LEARNING OBJECTIVES

At the end of the session the student should be able to:

1. Describe ultrastructure of basement membrane.
2. Describe ultrastructure of cilia.
3. Describe ultrastructure of microvilli.
4. Describe ultrastructure of stereocilia.

I. ULTRASTRUCTURE OF BASEMENT MEMBRANE

1. Name the layers of basement membrane as seen under the electron microscope.

_____

_____

_____

_____

_____

_____

_____

2. Write two functions of basement membrane.

_____

_____

_____

_____

_____

_____

_____

_____

_____

Date:

II. ULTRASTRUCTURE OF CILIA

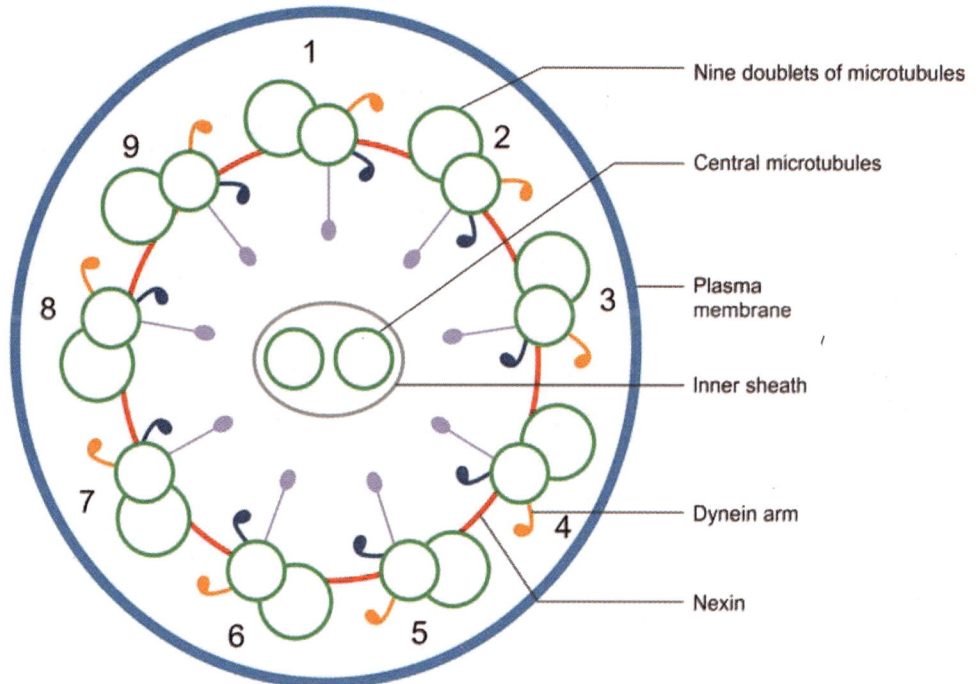

1. Describe the structure of cilia as seen under the electron microscope.

_____

_____

_____

_____

2. Write two functions of cilia.

_____

_____

_____

3. Draw ultrastructure diagram of cilia.

Date:

III. ULTRASTRUCTURE OF MICROVILLI

1. Microvilli are folds of cell membrane that extend outwards from the surface of cell.
2. They are found in organs like GIT for absorption. They increase the area of cell membrane.
3. Microvilli do not move, unlike cilia.
4. Microvilli have actin filaments running parallel to each other down the length of microvilli.
5. The actin filaments are bound to the plasma membrane by supporting proteins.

1. Describe the structure of microvilli as seen under the electron microscope.

_____

_____

_____

_____

_____

_____

_____

_____

2. Write two functions of microvilli.

_____

_____

_____

_____

_____

_____

_____

3. Write the differences between cilia and microvilli

	Cilia	Microvilli
Length		
Diameter		
Motility		
Pattern of microtubules		
Function		
For example		

Date:

ULTRASTRUCTURE OF STEREOCILIA

1. Stereocilia have actin filaments, cross links of fimbrin and espin, and myosin.
2. Stereocilia taper at their bases with diminishing actin filaments.
3. Actin filaments extend into the cuticular plate which a rigid platform formed by a meshwork of actin filaments.
4. Interciliary links are present at tip and laterally.
5. Stereocilia respond as a unit and move as rigid rods pivoting at their insertion.

1. Describe the structure of stereocilia as seen under the electron microscope.

_____

_____

_____

_____

_____

_____

2. Write two functions of stereocilia.

_____

_____

_____

_____

3. Where are stereocilia found?

_____

_____

_____

_____

Date:

SDL NOTES

Date:

SDL NOTES

Date:

COMPONENTS OF CONNECTIVE TISSUE PROPER

• Name the cells found in connective tissue:

_____

_____

_____

_____

Fibres of Connective Tissue

Collagen fibres are thick, wavy and do not branch. They appear pink with H & E staining.

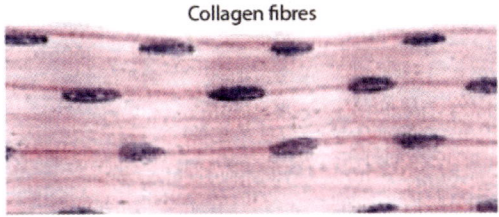

Collagen fibres

Elastic fibres are thin and straight with branching present in individual fibres. They appear pink with H & E staining.

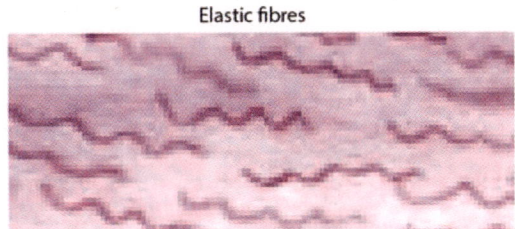

Elastic fibres

Reticular fibres are thin and form a network. They cannot be seen with H & E stain and require special staining (silver staining) where they stain black.

Date:

LOOSE AREOLAR TISSUE

SPECIFIC LEARNING OBJECTIVES

At the end of the session the student should be able to:

1. Identify loose areolar tissue under light microscope.
2. Give their distribution.
3. Write their functions.
4. Draw a diagram of microanatomy of loose areolar tissue.

Distribution and function

_____

_____

_____

_____

Three points of identification

_____

_____

_____

_____

_____

_____

Date:

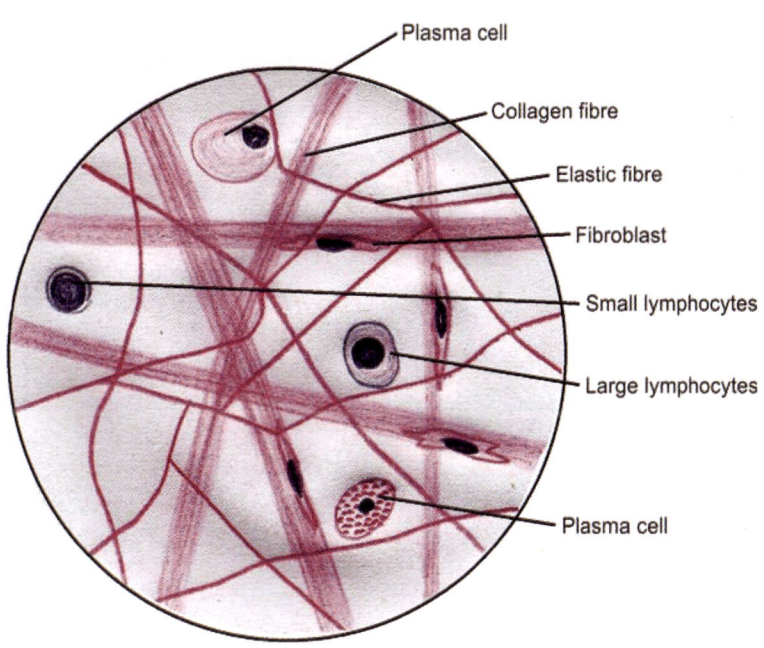

- Plasma cell
- Collagen fibre
- Elastic fibre
- Fibroblast
- Small lymphocytes
- Large lymphocytes
- Plasma cell

Date:

DENSE REGULAR CONNECTIVE TISSUE (TENDON LS)

SPECIFIC LEARNING OBJECTIVES

At the end of the session the student should be able to:

1. Identify tendon (LS) under light microscope.
2. Describe the cells in dense regular connective tissue.
3. Describe the fibres in dense regular connective tissue.
4. Identify the nuclei in LS
5. Draw a diagram of microanatomy of dense regular connective tissue (tendon LS)

Distribution and function

_____

_____

_____

_____

Three points of identification

_____

_____

_____

_____

_____

_____

Date:

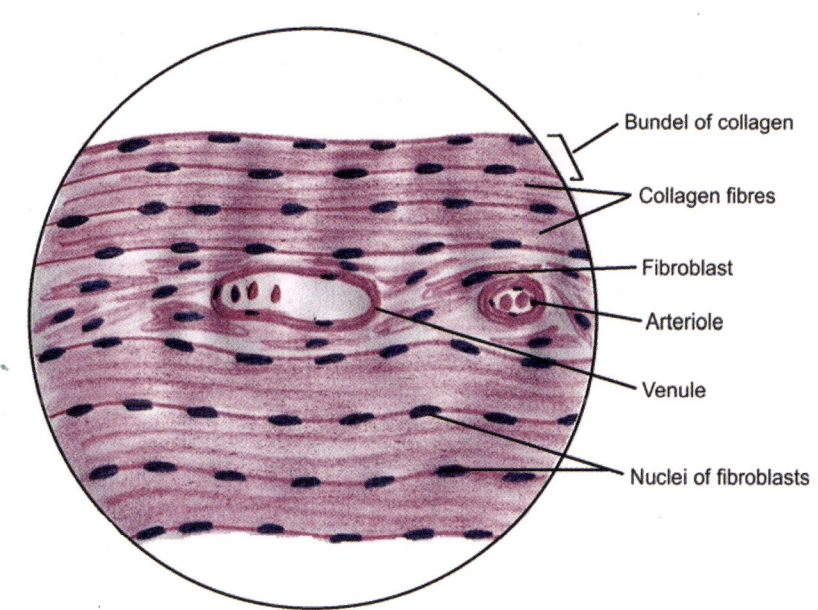

- Bundel of collagen
- Collagen fibres
- Fibroblast
- Arteriole
- Venule
- Nuclei of fibroblasts

Date:

DENSE REGULAR CONNECTIVE TISSUE (TENDON TS)

SPECIFIC LEARNING OBJECTIVES

At the end of the session the student should be able to:

1. Identify tendon (TS) under light microscope.
2. Identify the nuclei in TS
3. Draw a diagram of microanatomy of dense regular connective tissue (tendon TS)

Distribution and function

_____

_____

_____

_____

Three points of identification

_____

_____

_____

_____

_____

_____

Date:

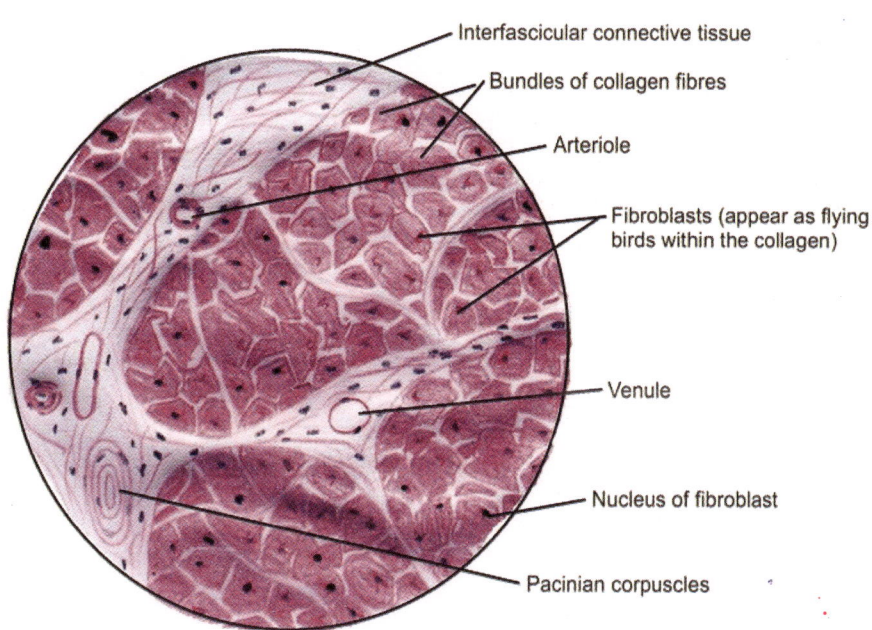

Interfascicular connective tissue

Bundles of collagen fibres

Arteriole

Fibroblasts (appear as flying
birds within the collagen)

Venule

Nucleus of fibroblast

Pacinian corpuscles

Date:

CONNECTIVE TISSUE HISTOLOGY

Number	Competency	Domain	Level	Core (Y/N)	Teaching/learning method	Assessment method	Number required to certify
AN 66.1	Describe and identify various types of connective tissue with functional correlation	K/S	SH	Y	Lecture, practical	Written/skill assessment	

SPECIFIC LEARNING OBJECTIVES

At the end of the session the student should be able to:
1. Classify connective tissue.
2. Name the components of connective tissue.
3. Name the three types of fibres in connective tissue.
4. Name the types of proper connective tissues with examples.

Classification of Connective Tissue

1. Ordinary
2. Loose areolar connective tissue, e.g. subperitoneal tissue, endomysium, lamina propria.
3. Dense collagenous
   a. Dense regular connective tissue, e.g. tendon, ligaments, aponeurosis
   b. Dense irregular connective tissue, e.g. reticular layer of dermis
4. Connective tissue with special properties
   a. Adipose, e.g. subcutaneous adipose tissue
   b. Mucoid, e.g. Wharton's jelly
   c. Reticular, e.g. stroma of lymphoid and myeloid (bone marrow) organs
   d. Elastic, e.g. blood vessels, ligamentum nuchae
   e. Scleral
      i. Cartilage
      ii. Bone
5. Lymphoid
6. Haemopoietic

Date:

SDL NOTES

Date:

SDL NOTES

Date:

ULTRASTRUCTURE OF CONNECTIVE TISSUE

Number	Competency	Domain	Level	Core (Y/N)	Teaching/learning method	Assessment method	Number required to certify
AN 66.2	Describe the ultrastructure of connective tissue	K	KH	N	Lecture, practical	Written	

SPECIFIC LEARNING OBJECTIVES

At the end of the session the student should be able to:

1. Describe the ultrastructure of ground substance of connective tissue.
2. Describe the ultrastructure of collagen fibres and their types.
3. Describe the ultrastructure of elastic fibres.
4. Describe the ultrastructure of reticular fibres.

GROUND SUBSTANCE

- Ground substance is made up of glycosaminoglycans (mucopolysaccharides), proteoglycans and glycoproteins and is a gel like substance.
- Different types of GAGs present are as follows: Chondroitin sulphate, hyaluronic acid, dermatan sulphate, heparin, heparan sulphate and keratan sulphate.
- They are long chain un-branched polysaccharides.
- Proteoglycans are large molecules with a core protein in the centre and numerous GAGs (except hyaluronic acid) attached around it.
  o Hyaluronic acid is bound to core protein through a link protein.
- Glycoproteins have oligosaccharide chains attached to them.
  o Types of glycoproteins: Fibronectin, laminin, entactin, osteonectin, chondronectin
  o Fibronectin helps in adhesion of cells to extracellular matrix (ECM).
  o Laminin helps in adhesion of epithelial cells to basement membrane (BM).
  o Entactin binds laminin type IV collagen to BM.
  o Osteonectin is present in bone and helps in bone mineralization
  o Chondronectin is present in cartilages and helps in adhesion of chondrocytes to ECM.

FIBRES

- Fibres are formed by fibroblasts and are of 3 types: Collagen, elastic, reticular.
- Collagen fibres provide tensile strength. Collagen fibres are eosinophilic and appear pink on H & E stain. Some types of collagen present in body are as follows:
  o Type I: Presents in fascia, tendon, ligaments, etc.
  o Type II: Presents in hyaline cartilage
  o Type III: Presents in reticular fibres
  o Type IV: Presents in basement membrane
- Elastic fibres can stretch and so provide elasticity. They are made of elastin protein and microfibrils.
  o They are thinner than collagen fibres and show branching.
  o They are eosinophilic and have the property to recoil.
- Reticular fibres form a network for framework in lymph nodes, spleen, bone marrow, basement membrane, etc.
  o They are not stained by H & E stain.

Date:

CELLS

Fibroblasts

- Active fibroblasts appear branched and have a large ovoid nucleus in the centre.
- Inactive fibroblasts are smaller and spindle shaped and have a flat nucleus. They are called fibrocytes.

Fibroblast

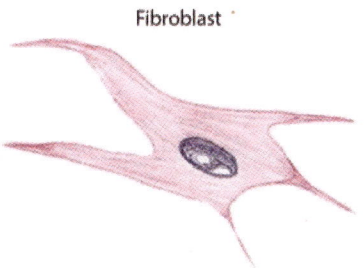

Adipocyte

- It is round in shape and during histological section the fat droplet is lost. Therefore, on staining only a thin rim of cytoplasm is visible.
- Nucleus is flattened and eccentric. Appearance of the cell is like that of a signet ring.

Adipocyte
Peripheral rim of cytoplasm

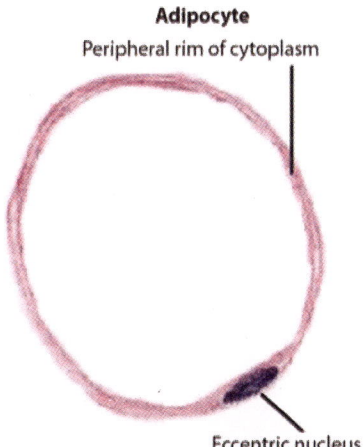

Eccentric nucleus

Date:

SDL NOTES

Date:

SDL NOTES

Date:

CARTILAGE

Number	Competency	Domain	Level	Core (Y/N)	Teaching/learning method	Assessment method	Number required to certify
AN 71.2	Identify cartilage under the microscope and describe various types and structure–function correlation of the same	K/S	SH	Y	Lecture, practical	Written/skill assessment	

SPECIFIC LEARNING OBJECTIVES

At the end of the session the student should be able to:
1. Name the components of cartilage.
2. Classify cartilage

Components of Cartilage

- Cells—chondrocytes (large cells with round euchromatic nucleus, granular and basophilic cytoplasm), chondroblasts (small, flat, irregular shape with branching processes). Cells are present in lacunae and take basic stain.
- Intercellular substance is composed of collagen or elastic fibres and ground substance. The ground substance is basophilic.

Classification of Cartilage

1. Hyaline cartilage
2. Elastic cartilage
3. Fibrocartilage

STRUCTURE OF CARTILAGE

Perichondrium

- It consists of two layers: Outer fibrous and inner chondrogenic.
- Perichondrium has blood supply, nerve supply and lymphatics as compared to cartilage which does not have these.

Cartilage

- There is extracellular matrix in which cells are embedded.
- Chondroblasts are oval in shape and present in the periphery. They are precursors of chondrocytes.
- Chondrocytes are oval near the periphery and round in deeper area. They lie within lacunae. ECM is secreted by chondrocytes.
- Matrix is basophilic. It has type II collagen which has the same refractive index as that of the ground substance, therefore, the fibres cannot be distinguished and the matrix appears homogenous in hyaline cartilage.
- Elastic fibres are eosinophilic in H & E stain and are present in addition to the matrix in elastic cartilage.
- Fibrocartilage does not have a perichondrium. It has Type I collagen fibres running parallel in ground substance. Chondrocytes are arranged in rows between layers of collagen, within the lacunae.

Date:

Answer the Following

1. What is territorial matrix?
2. What is inter-territorial matrix?
3. Why does the matrix of hyaline cartilage appear homogenous?
4. What type of cartilage is present in the following?

Tissue	Cartilage	Tissue	Cartilage
Trachea		Bronchus	
Nasal cartilage		Costal cartilage	
Articular cartilage		Epiphyseal cartilage	
Thyroid cartilage		Cricoid cartilage	
Basal part of arytenoid cartilage		Epiglottis	
External ear		External acoustic meatus	
Pharyngotympanic tube		Apical part of arytenoid cartilage	
Corniculate cartilage		Cuneiform cartilage	
Intervertebral disc		Articular disc of joints	

Date:

SDL NOTES

Date:

SDL NOTES

Date:

HYALINE CARTILAGE

SPECIFIC LEARNING OBJECTIVES

At the end of the session the student should be able to:

1. Identify hyaline cartilage under light microscope.
2. Identify perichondrium and chondrocytes under light microscope.
3. Describe the appearance of ground substance under light microscope and give reason for such appearance.
4. Give examples of tissues with hyaline cartilage.
5. Draw a diagram of microanatomy of hyaline cartilage.

Distribution and function

_____

_____

_____

_____

Three points of identification

_____

_____

_____

_____

_____

_____

Date:

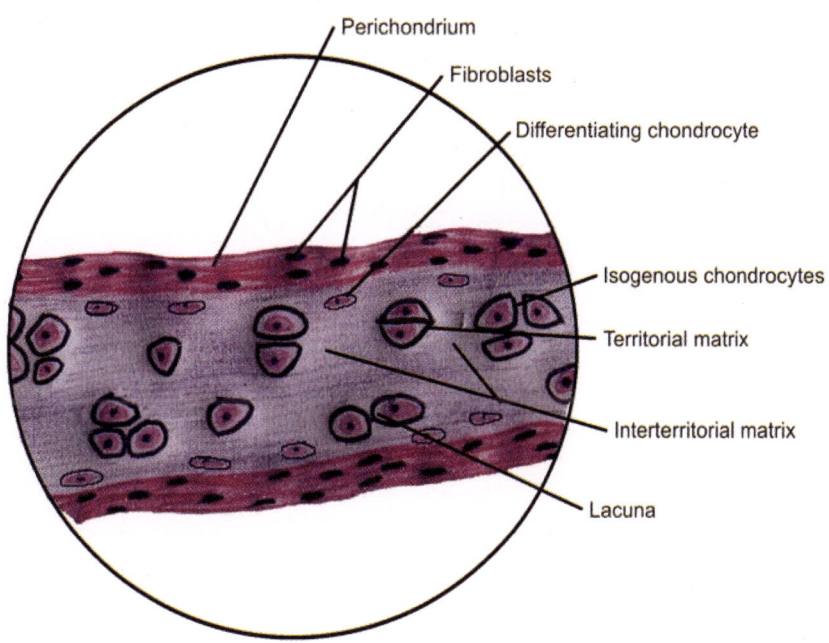

Date:

ELASTIC CARTILAGE

SPECIFIC LEARNING OBJECTIVES

At the end of the session the student should be able to:

1. Identify elastic cartilage under light microscope.
2. Identify perichondrium and chondrocytes under light microscope.
3. Identify elastic fibres.
4. Draw a diagram of microanatomy of elastic cartilage.

Distribution and function

_____

_____

_____

_____

Three points of identification

_____

_____

_____

_____

_____

_____

Date:

Perichondrium

Fibrocytes of perichondrium

Chondrogenic layer

Lacunae with chondrocytes

Cartilage matrix with elastic fibres

Nuclei of chondrocytes

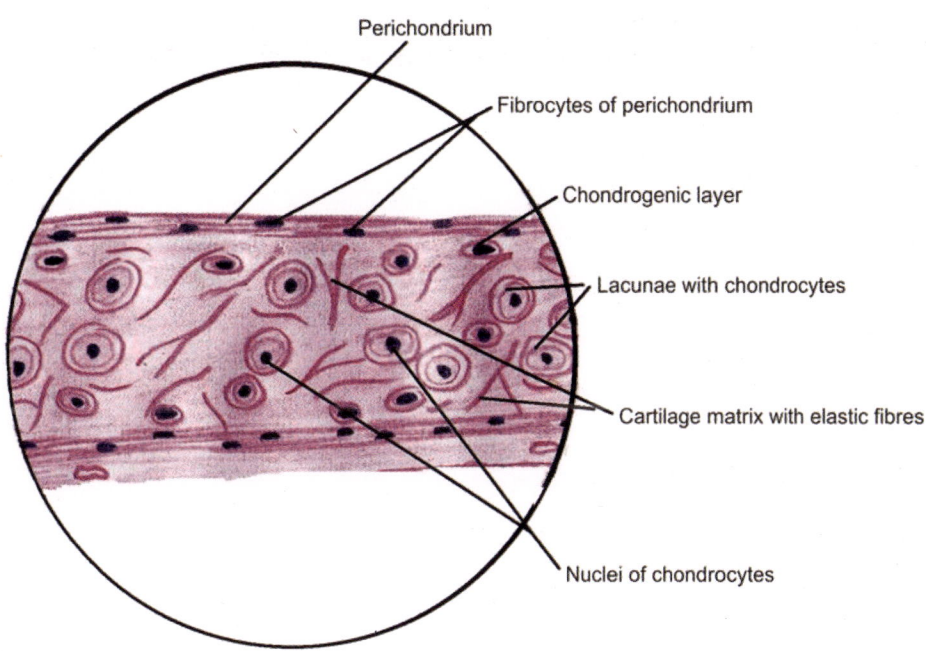

Date:

FIBROCARTILAGE

SPECIFIC LEARNING OBJECTIVES

At the end of the session the student should be able to:
1. Identify fibrocartilage under light microscope.
2. Identify chondrocytes under light microscope.
3. Give examples of fibrocartilage.
4. Draw a diagram of microanatomy of fibrocartilage.

Distribution and function

_____

_____

_____

_____

Three points of identification

_____

_____

_____

_____

_____

_____

Date:

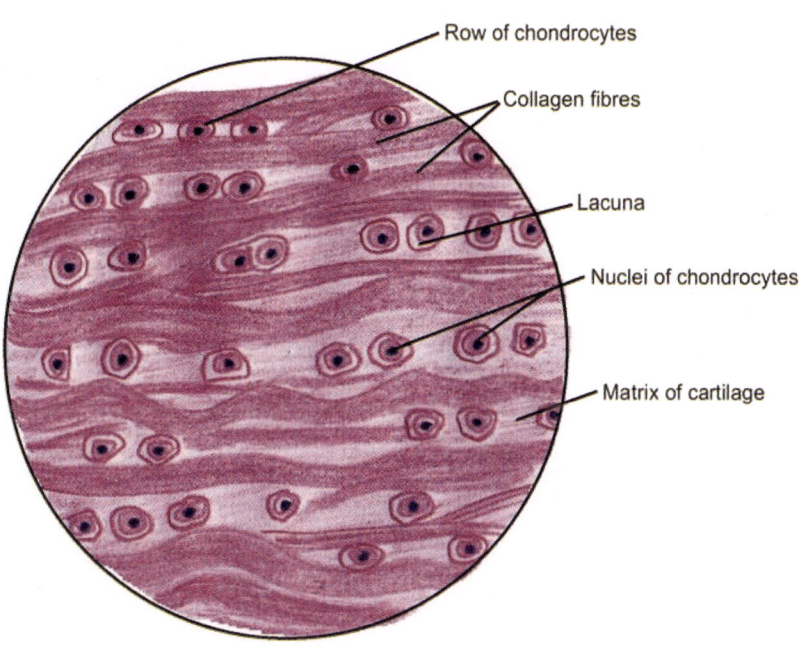

Row of chondrocytes

Collagen fibres

Lacuna

Nuclei of chondrocytes

Matrix of cartilage

Date:

SDL NOTES

Date:

SDL NOTES

Date:

<table>
<tr><th>Number</th><th>Competency</th><th>Domain</th><th>Level</th><th>Core (Y/N)</th><th>Teaching/learning method</th><th>Assessment method</th><th>Number required to certify</th></tr>
<tr><td>AN 71.1</td><td>Identify bone under the microscope; classify various types and describe structure-function correlation of the same</td><td>K/S</td><td>SH</td><td>Y</td><td>Lecture, practical</td><td>Written/skill assessment</td><td></td></tr>
</table>

SPECIFIC LEARNING OBJECTIVES

At the end of the session the student should be able to:
1. Identify and describe the features of an LS of compact bone.
2. Identify and describe the features of a TS of compact bone.
3. Describe Haversian system.
4. Identify and describe the features of a TS of spongy bone.
5. Describe the histological components of bone.

HISTOLOGICAL COMPONENTS OF BONE

- Periosteum covers outer surface of bone. It has two layers—outer fibrous layer of collagen fibres; and inner osteogenic layer having osteoprogenitor cells which form osteoblasts. Collagen fibres of outer layer binding the periosteum to bone are called Sharpey's fibres.
- Endosteum lines the inner surface of bone. It has a single layer of osteoprogenitor cells.
- Osteoprogenitor cells are irregular elongated cells having pale nucleus and a pale cytoplasm.
- Osteoblasts are large cells, cuboidal or low columnar, with cytoplasmic processes. They have intensely basophilic cytoplasm and round nucleus situated at one side of cytoplasm and prominent nucleolus. They synthesize collagen fibres and matrix of a bone.
- Osteocytes are flattened cells smaller than osteoblasts. They have processes that lie in canaliculi. Their cytoplasm is less basophilic. They are present in the lacunae of bones. They are resting living cells. They can convert to osteoblasts or osteoclasts.
- Osteoclasts are multinucleated giant cells with lightly basophilic or acidophilic cytoplasm. They are present on bone surfaces that are undergoing resorption. They lie in Howship's lacunae
- Ground substance has organic and inorganic elements.

HAVERSIAN SYSTEM (OSTEON) IN A COMPACT BONE

- Each haversian system has a central haversian canal (containing blood vessels and nerves), surrounded by 6–12 concentric haversian lamellae made up of collagen fibres and deposited calcium salts.
- There are interstitial lamellae between adjacent haversian lamellae.
- Outer circumferential lamellae lie just adjacent to the periosteum and inner circumferential lamellae lie next to the endosteum.
- Lacunae containing osteocytes are present between the lamellae. Lacunae communicate with each other by canaliculi which have cytoplasmic processes of osteocytes.
- Volkmann's canals connect haversian canals and marrow cavity with each other.

CANCELLOUS/SPONGY BONE

- Bone tissue is arranged in the form of thin plates called trabeculae. Bone marrow is present between the trabeculae.
- Haversian system is absent but osteocytes are present in lacunae.
- Osteoblasts and osteoclasts are present near the margins of trabeculae.

Date:

COMPACT BONE (TS)

SPECIFIC LEARNING OBJECTIVES

At the end of the session the student should be able to:

1. Identify compact bone in TS under a light microscope.
2. Identify its component cells, haversian system and fibres.
3. Draw a diagram of microanatomy of compact bone (TS)

Distribution and function

_____

_____

_____

_____

Three points of identification

_____

_____

_____

_____

_____

_____

Date:

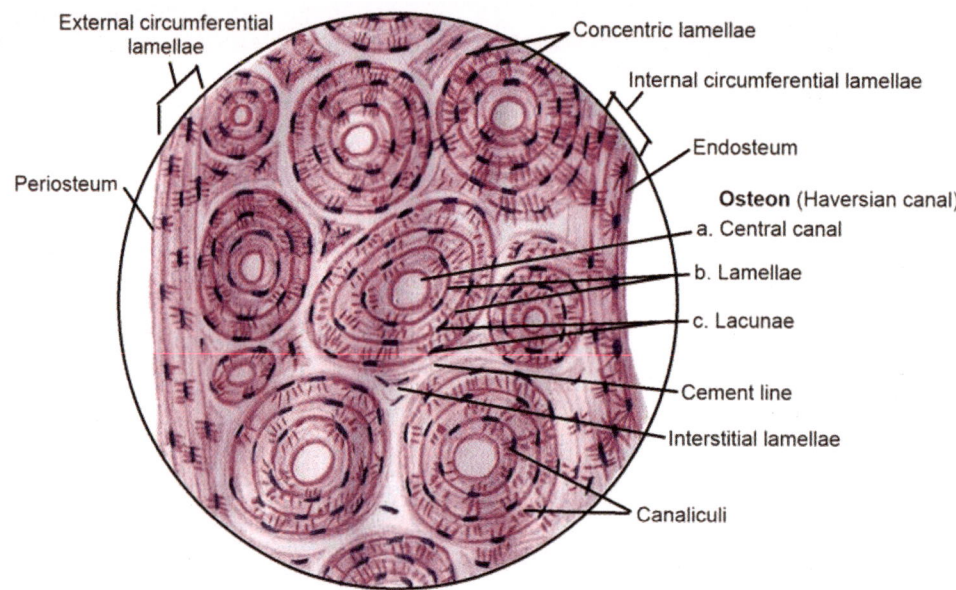

External circumferential lamellae

Concentric lamellae

Internal circumferential lamellae

Endosteum

Periosteum

Osteon (Haversian canal)
a. Central canal
b. Lamellae
c. Lacunae

Cement line

Interstitial lamellae

Canaliculi

Date:

COMPACT BONE (LS)

SPECIFIC LEARNING OBJECTIVES

At the end of the session the student should be able to:

1. Identify compact bone in LS under light microscope.
2. Identify haversian and Volkmann's canals.
3. Draw a diagram of microanatomy of compact bone (LS).

Distribution and function

_____

_____

_____

_____

Three points of identification

_____

_____

_____

_____

_____

_____

Date:

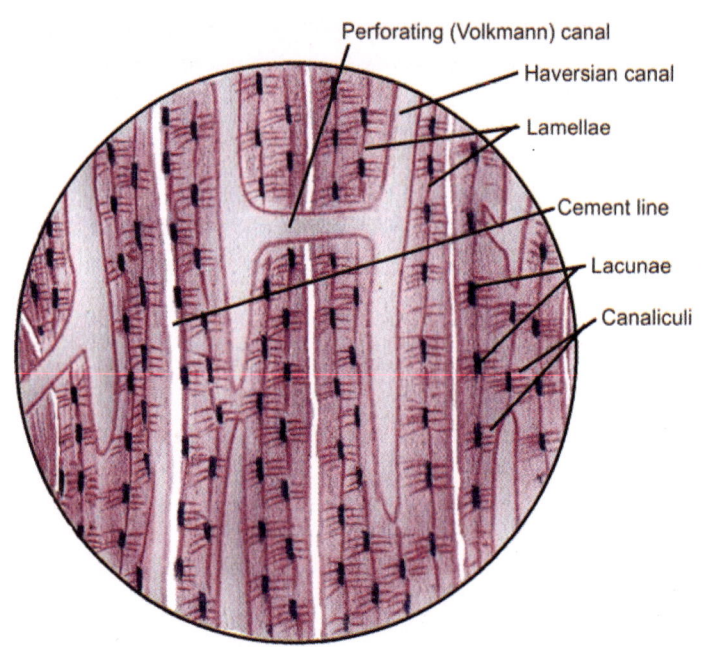

Perforating (Volkmann) canal
Haversian canal
Lamellae
Cement line
Lacunae
Canaliculi

Date:

CANCELLOUS BONE (SPONGY BONE) TS

SPECIFIC LEARNING OBJECTIVES

At the end of the session the student should be able to:

1. Identify cancellous bone under light microscope.
2. Identify trabeculae and bone marrow under light microscope.
3. Draw a diagram showing microanatomy of cancellous bone (TS).

Distribution and function

_____

_____

_____

_____

Three points of identification

_____

_____

_____

_____

_____

_____

Date:

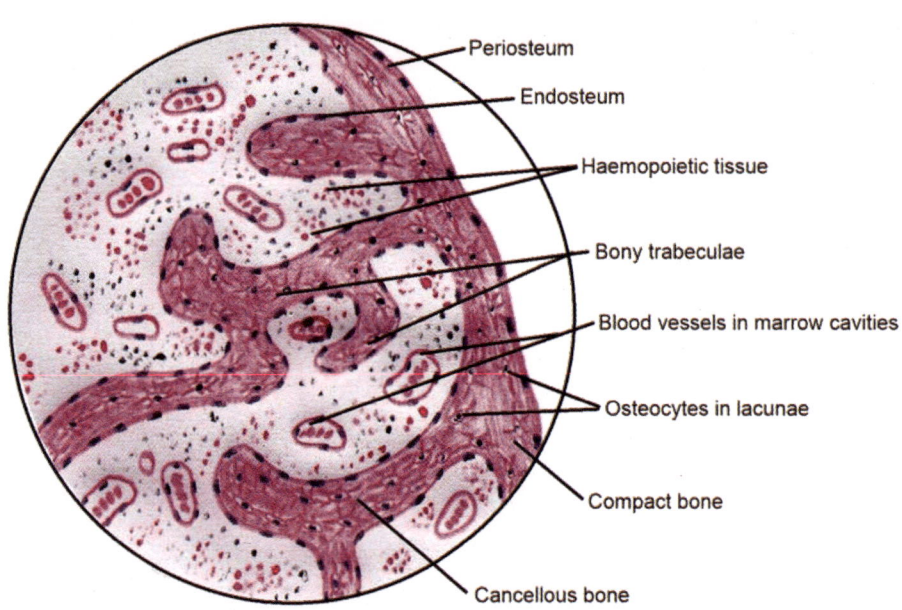

- Periosteum
- Endosteum
- Haemopoietic tissue
- Bony trabeculae
- Blood vessels in marrow cavities
- Osteocytes in lacunae
- Compact bone
- Cancellous bone

Date:

SDL NOTES

Date:

SDL NOTES

Date:

MUSCULAR TISSUE

Number	Competency	Domain	Level	Core (Y/N)	Teaching/learning method	Assessment method	Number required to certify
AN 67.1	Describe and identify various types of muscle under the microscope	K/S	SH	Y	Lecture, practical	Written/skill assessment	

SKELETAL MUSCLE (STRIATED, SOMATIC, STRIPED, VOLUNTARY)

- Muscle fibres are long, cylindrical and multinucleated. Nuclei are present at the periphery.
- Each fibre is covered by endomysium. Many muscle fibres are held together as fascicles. Each fasciculus is surrounded by epimysium. Whole skeletal muscle is surrounded by perimysium.
- Muscle fibres have transverse and longitudinal striations. There are alternate light (I) and dark (A) bands in transverse striations.
- There are neuromuscular spindles within the skeletal muscle.

SMOOTH MUSCLE (UNSTRIPED, INVOLUNTARY, UNSTRIATED)

- Muscle fibres are bundles of spindle shaped cells with centrally placed oval nucleus.
- Transverse striations are absent.

CARDIAC MUSCLE

- Cardiac muscle fibres show branching and anastomoses. Their nuclei are oval and centrally placed.
- There are transverse striations, though not as prominent as skeletal muscles.
- They show intercalated discs which are junctional complexes where the ends of individual muscle fibres join.

Date:

SKELETAL MUSCLE (LS)

SPECIFIC LEARNING OBJECTIVES

At the end of the session the student should be able to:

1. Identify LS of skeletal muscle under light microscope.
2. Identify microscopic features of skeletal muscle.
3. Draw a diagram of microanatomy of skeletal muscle (LS).

Distribution and function

_____

_____

_____

_____

Three points of identification

_____

_____

_____

_____

_____

_____

Date:

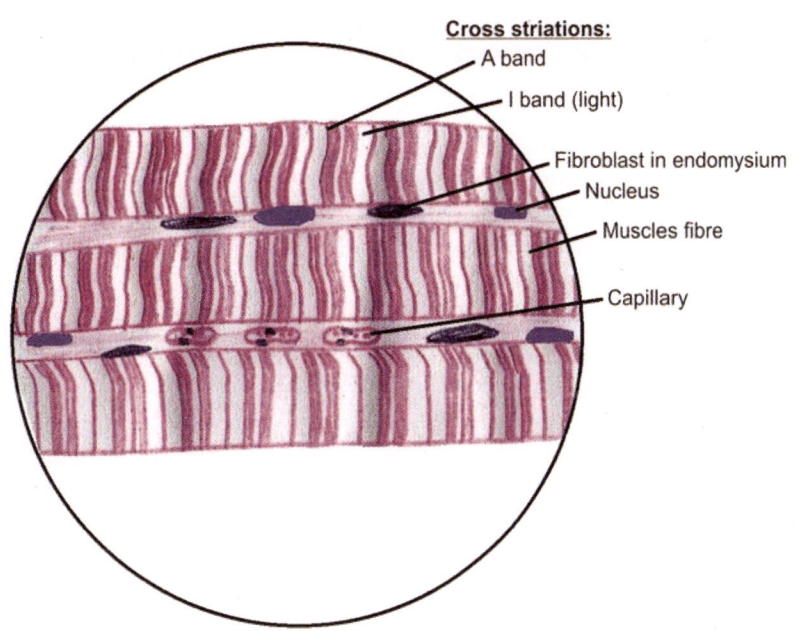

Cross striations:
- A band
- I band (light)
- Fibroblast in endomysium
- Nucleus
- Muscles fibre
- Capillary

Date:

SKELETAL MUSCLE (TS)

SPECIFIC LEARNING OBJECTIVES

At the end of the session the student should be able to:

1. Identify TS of skeletal muscle under light microscope.
2. Identify where the nuclei are present in TS.
3. Identify endomysium, epimysium, perimysium.
4. Draw a diagram of microanatomy of skeletal muscle (TS).

Distribution and function

_____

_____

_____

_____

Three points of identification

_____

_____

_____

_____

_____

_____

Date:

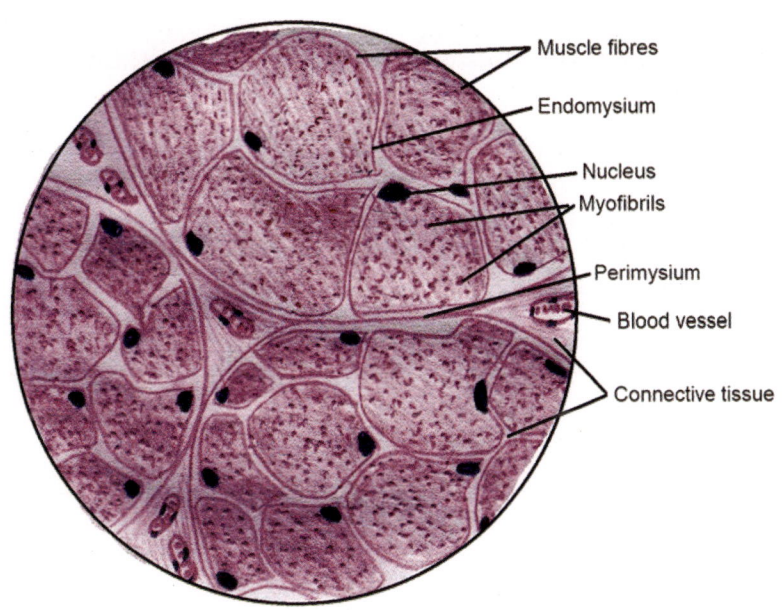

Muscle fibres

Endomysium

Nucleus

Myofibrils

Perimysium

Blood vessel

Connective tissue

Date:

CARDIAC MUSCLE (LS)

SPECIFIC LEARNING OBJECTIVES

At the end of the session the student should be able to:

1. Identify LS of cardiac muscle under light microscope.
2. Identify where the nuclei are present in LS.
3. Identify branching and anastomosing of muscle fibres and intercalated discs.
4. Draw a diagram of microanatomy of LS of cardiac muscle.

Function

Three points of identification

Date:

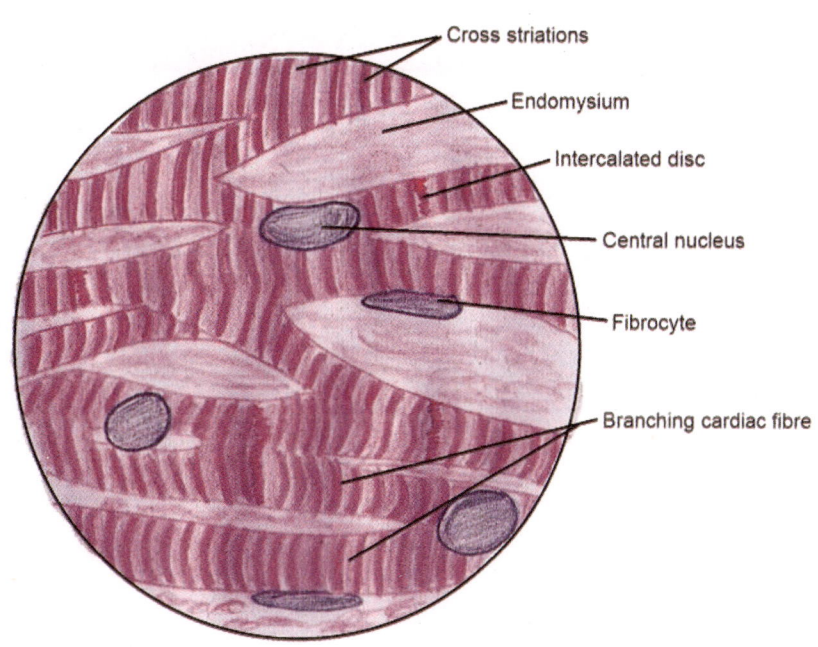

Cross striations

Endomysium

Intercalated disc

Central nucleus

Fibrocyte

Branching cardiac fibre

Date:

SMOOTH MUSCLE (LS)

SPECIFIC LEARNING OBJECTIVES

At the end of the session the student should be able to:

1. Identify LS of smooth muscle under light microscope.
2. Identify where the nuclei are present in LS.
3. Draw a diagram of microanatomy of LS of smooth muscle.

Distribution and function

_____

_____

_____

_____

Three points of identification

_____

_____

_____

_____

_____

Date:

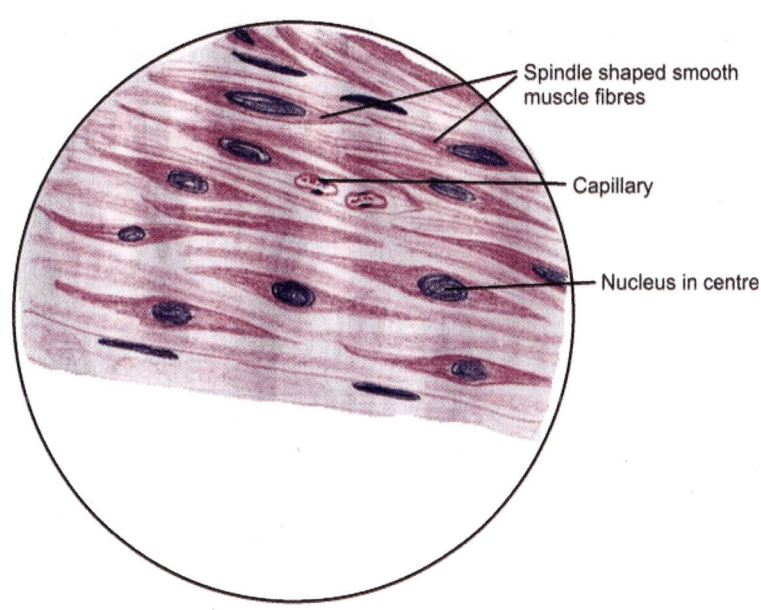

Spindle shaped smooth muscle fibres

Capillary

Nucleus in centre

Date:

SMOOTH MUSCLE (TS)

SPECIFIC LEARNING OBJECTIVES

At the end of the session the student should be able to:

1. Identify TS of smooth muscle under light microscope.
2. Identify where the nuclei are present in TS.
3. Draw a diagram of microanatomy of TS. of smooth muscle.

Distribution and function

_____

_____

_____

_____

Three points of identification

_____

_____

_____

_____

_____

_____

Date:

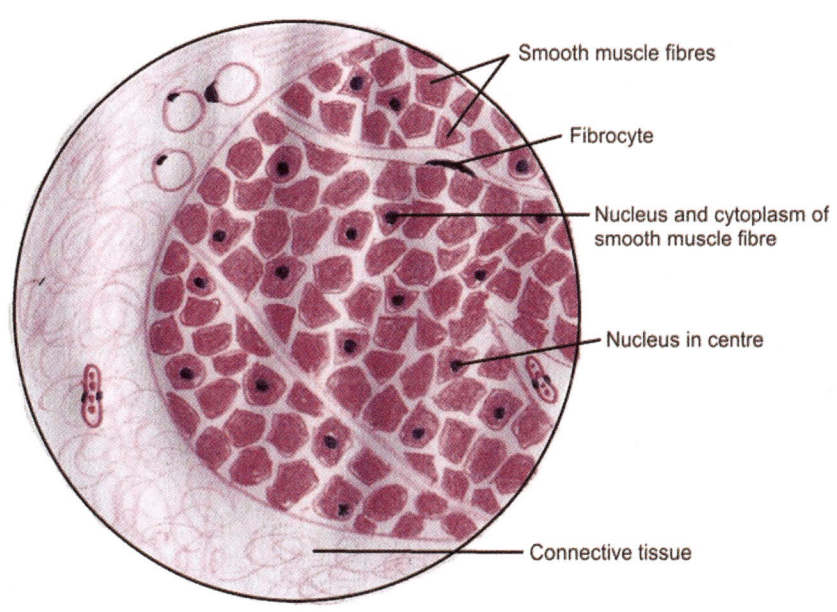

- Smooth muscle fibres
- Fibrocyte
- Nucleus and cytoplasm of smooth muscle fibre
- Nucleus in centre
- Connective tissue

Date:

SDL NOTES

Date:

SDL NOTES

Date:

MUSCLE (ULTRASTRUCTURE)

Number	Competency	Domain	Level	Core (Y/N)	Teaching/learning method	Assessment method	Number required to certify
AN 67.2	Classify muscle and describe the structure-function correlation of the same	K/S	SH	Y	Lecture, practical	Written	
AN 67.3	Describe the ultrastructure of muscular tissue	K	KH	N	Lecture, practical	Written	

SPECIFIC LEARNING OBJECTIVES

At the end of the session the student should be able to:
1. Classify muscle.
2. Correlate function with structure of muscle.
3. Describe ultrastructure of skeletal muscle.
4. Describe ultrastructure of smooth muscle.
5. Describe ultrastructure of cardiac muscle.

Answer the Following

Skeletal Muscle

1. Alternate light and dark bands in myofibrils are caused by a difference in the

_____

2. Dark band is known as _____ band (anisotropic).

3. Light band is known as _____ band (isotropic).

4. A band possesses a light zone called _____ line or Hensen's line. In the middle of this light zone there is a dark line called _____ line.

5. I band has a dark line dividing it known as _____ line or _____ membrane.

6. There are 2 types of myofilaments in a myofibril known as_____ and _____.

7. Sarcomere is a unit of contraction and lies between two _____ lines.

8. Draw a schematic diagram of ultrastructure of a sarcomere.

Date:

9. Describe the contraction of a skeletal muscle in correlation with its ultrastructure.

_____

_____

_____

_____

_____

_____

_____

_____

_____

_____

Cardiac Muscle

1. Cardiac muscle has more _____ than skeletal muscle.

2. Draw the ultrastructure of intercalated disc of cardiac muscle.

3. T tubules are _____ in smooth muscles.

4. Myofilaments are arranged obliquely in the muscle cells. Due to this arrangement contraction causes formation of blebs of cell membrane which disappear when muscle relaxes.

5. The thin filament of smooth muscle is composed of actin and tropomyosin. There is no _____.

Date:

SDL NOTES

Date:

SDL NOTES

Date:

NERVOUS TISSUE

Number	Competency	Domain	Level	Core (Y/N)	Teaching/learning method	Assessment method	Number required to certify
AN68.1	Describe and identify multipolar and unipolar neuron, ganglia, peripheral nerve	K/S	SH	Y	Lecture, practical	Written/skill assessment	
AN68.2	Describe the structure-function correlation of neuron	K	SH	Y	Lecture, practical	Written	
AN68.3	Describe the ultrastructure of nervous tissue	K	SH	Y	Lecutre, practical	Written	

Types of neurons on the basis of cell body processes

1. **Multipolar neuron:** It has more than one dendrite. For example, cell bodies of multipolar neurons present in autonomic ganglia. The cell bodies appear large (but smaller than cell bodies in dorsal root ganglia) with large nucleus which lies eccentrically.

2. **Unipolar/pseudounipolar neuron:** On light microscopy the cell bodies (which are present in spinal/dorsal root ganglia) appear as large cells with large nucleus and prominent large nucleolus.

The nerve fibres of these neurons lie in peripheral nerves which may be myelinated or unmyelinated. Since the cell bodies containing the nucleus of neuron lie in the ganglia, nerve fibres do not have nuclei. The nuclei that may be seen on TS or LS of peripheral nerve are those of Schwann cells or fibroblasts.

ULTRASTRUCTURE OF NEURON

- Cell body (perikaryon) is polygonal. It has nucleus and perinuclear cytoplasm. Nucleus is large, spherical and centrally placed with a single prominent nucleolus and finely dispersed chromatin.
- Cytoplasm has abundant RER, polyribosomes, Nissl bodies, numerous SER, Golgi bodies, many mitochondria which are most abundant in axon terminal. There is extensive cytoskeleton for axonal transport.
- There is only one centriole—so they do not undergo cell divisions.

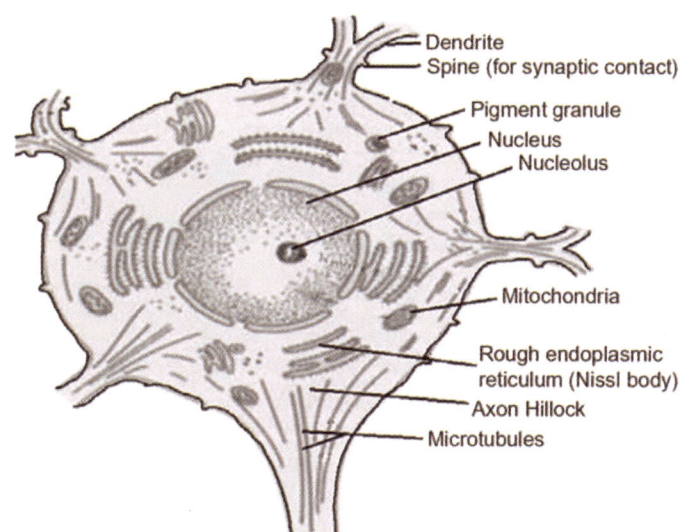

Axon

It originates from axon hillock. It is devoid of ribosome. Its dilated distal portion is called axon terminal and further there are end bulbs which participate in synapse.

Dendrites

They are multiple cytoplasmic processes from the cell body.

Date:

1. Draw the ultrastucture of body of neuron

2. Draw a longitudinal section of ultrastructure of myelinated nerve fibres

Date:

PERIPHERAL NERVE (TS)

SPECIFIC LEARNING OBJECTIVES

At the end of the session the student should be able to:

1. Identify TS of a peripheral nerve under light microscope.
2. Identify the epineurium, perineurium and endoneurium.
3. Explain what myelin sheath looks like in H & E stain.
4. Draw a diagram of microstructure of TS of a peripheral nerve.

Distribution and function of Schwann cells

_____

_____

_____

_____

Three points of identification

_____

_____

_____

_____

_____

_____

Date:

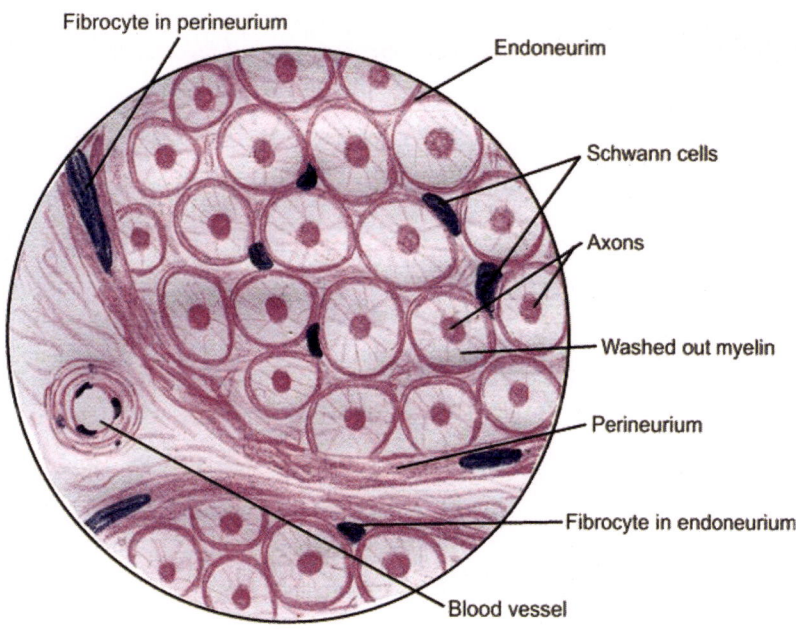

Fibrocyte in perineurium

Endoneurim

Schwann cells

Axons

Washed out myelin

Perineurium

Fibrocyte in endoneurium

Blood vessel

Date:

SENSORY/SPINAL/DORSAL ROOT GANGLION

SPECIFIC LEARNING OBJECTIVES

At the end of the session the student should be able to:

1. Identify a dorsal root ganglion under light microscope.
2. Identify the cell bodies of neurons and satellite cells.
3. Appreciate the clusters of cell bodies.
4. Identify whether it is unipolar or multipolar neuron.
5. Draw a diagram of microstructure of sensory ganglion.

Distribution and function

_____

_____

_____

_____

Three points of identification

_____

_____

_____

_____

_____

_____

Date:

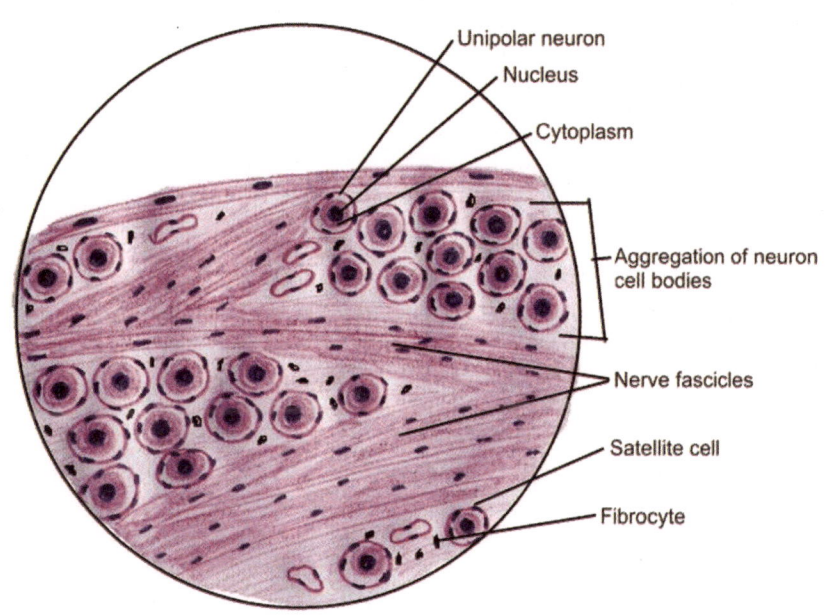

Unipolar neuron

Nucleus

Cytoplasm

Aggregation of neuron cell bodies

Nerve fascicles

Satellite cell

Fibrocyte

Date:

AUTONOMIC/SYMPATHETIC/PARASYMPATHETIC GANGLION

SPECIFIC LEARNING OBJECTIVES

At the end of the session the student should be able to:

1. Identify sympathetic ganglion under the light microscope.
2. Identify the multipolar neuron bodies.
3. Appreciate the wide spacing between cell bodies.
4. Appreciate the lesser number of satellite cells.
5. Draw the microstructure of an autonomic ganglion.

Distribution and function

_____

_____

_____

_____

Three points of identification

_____

_____

_____

_____

_____

_____

Date:

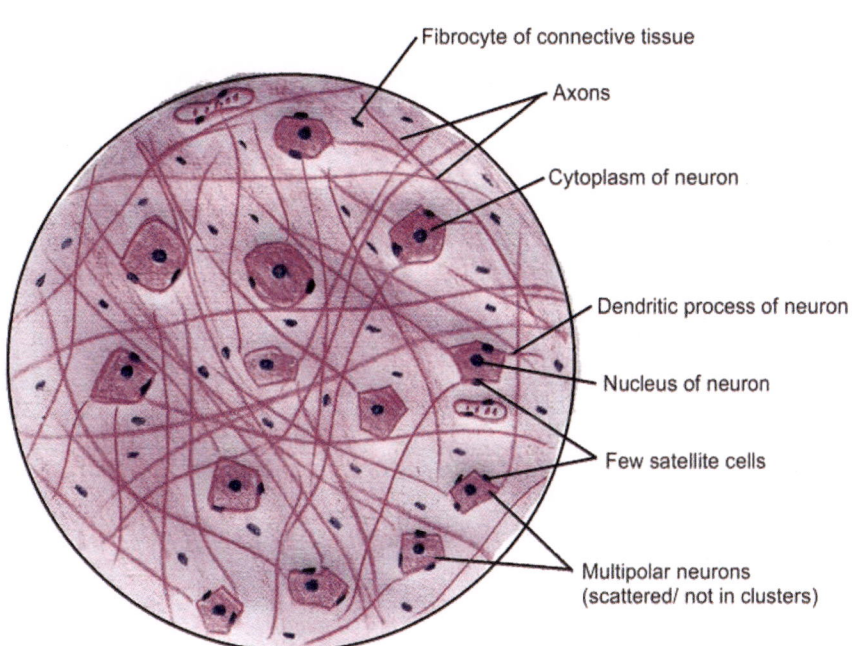

- Fibrocyte of connective tissue
- Axons
- Cytoplasm of neuron
- Dendritic process of neuron
- Nucleus of neuron
- Few satellite cells
- Multipolar neurons (scattered/ not in clusters)

Date:

SDL NOTES

Date:

SDL NOTES

Date:

EXOCRINE (SALIVARY) GLANDS HISTOLOGY

Number	Competency	Domain	Level	Core (Y/N)	Teaching/learning method	Assessment method	Number required to certify
AN 70.1	Identify exocrine gland under the microscope and distinguish between serous, mucous and mixed acini	K/S	SH	Y	Lecture, practical	Written/skill assessment	

CLASSIFICATION BASED ON TYPE OF SECRETION

1. Mucous glands
2. Serous glands
3. Mixed glands

MICROSCOPIC STRUCTURE OF EXOCRINE GLANDS

- **Parenchyma:** It consists of secretory cells. Shape of secretory units of salivary glands is acinar (round or oval). Therefore, there are serous, mucous or mixed acini depending upon the type of salivary gland.
- **Stroma:** It consists of connective tissue dividing the gland into lobules, lobes or forming its capsule. Blood vessels pass through the connective tissue.
- **Ducts:** Intralobular, interlobular, interlobar
- Myoepithelial cells are present in close relation to the secretory elements. They are stellate or fusiform in shape and lie between the secretory cells and basement membrane.

ACINI

- **Mucous acini:** They contain mucopolysaccharide secretion which does not stain with H & E stain. Therefore, the cells of mucous acini appear empty. The secretions near the apices push the nuclei towards the base of cells (near the basement membrane) making them appear flattened. There is a lumen in the centre of acinus which is larger as compared to that of serous acinous, e.g. sublingual salivary gland.
- **Serous acini:** Cells are triangular with round nucleus placed centrally/basal. Secretions are proteinous, therefore, the cytoplasm is granular and stains bluish with H & E. There are basal striations present in active cells in higher magnification. Lumen is small, e.g. Parotid gland.
- **Mixed acini:** Submandibular gland is a mixed salivary gland having both serous and mucous acini. Demilunes are present on mucous acini.

Demilunes of Gianuzzi

The mucous cells form tubules, but their ends are capped by serous cells, which constitute the serous demilunes. Under the light microscope the serous demilunes appear as semilunar dark stained caps on the light stained mucous acini. The demilunes are connected with the lumen of mucous acini by microscopic canaliculi to the lumen of acini. So the serous secretion of demilunes makes the secretion of mucous acini less viscid.

Ducts

- **Intercalated ducts:** Lined by cuboidal epithelium, are present in the lobules.
- **Striated ducts:** Formed by joining of several intercalated ducts. They are lined by simple columnar cells and have basal striations formed by folding of basal cell membrane. They have a larger lumen than intercalated ducts.
- **Interlobular ducts:** The epithelium varies from low columnar in smaller ducts to pseudostratified or stratified columnar epithelium in larger ducts.

ACTIVITY

1. Draw a well labelled single mucous acinus at high magnification in H & E staining.
2. Draw a well labelled single serous acinus at high magnification in H & E staining.
3. Draw a well labelled single mucous acinus with serous demilune at high magnification in H & E staining.
4. Draw a well labelled intercalated duct at high magnification in H & E staining.
5. Draw a well labelled striated duct at high magnification in H & E staining.
6. Draw a well labelled interlobular duct (striated or tall columnar) at high magnification in H & E staining.

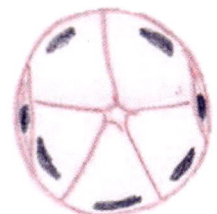   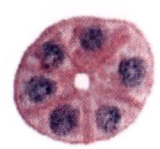   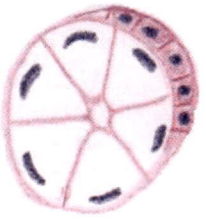

Mucous Acinus	**Serous Acinus**	**Mucous Acinus with Serous Demilune**

   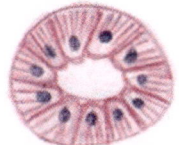   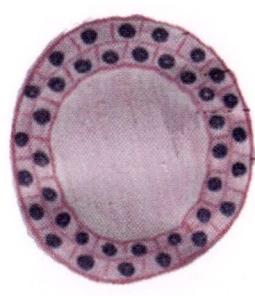

Intercalated Duct	**Striated Duct**	**Interlobular Duct**

Date:

SUBLINGUAL SALIVARY GLAND (MUCOUS GLAND)

SPECIFIC LEARNING OBJECTIVES

At the end of the session the student should be able to:

1. Identify mucous gland under light microscope.
2. Identify the mucous acini, ducts, connective tissue.
3. Explain what mucous looks like in H & E stain and why.
4. Draw the microstructure of microanatomy of sublingual/mucous salivary gland.

Function of mucous glands

_____

_____

_____

_____

Three points of identification

_____

_____

_____

_____

_____

_____

Date:

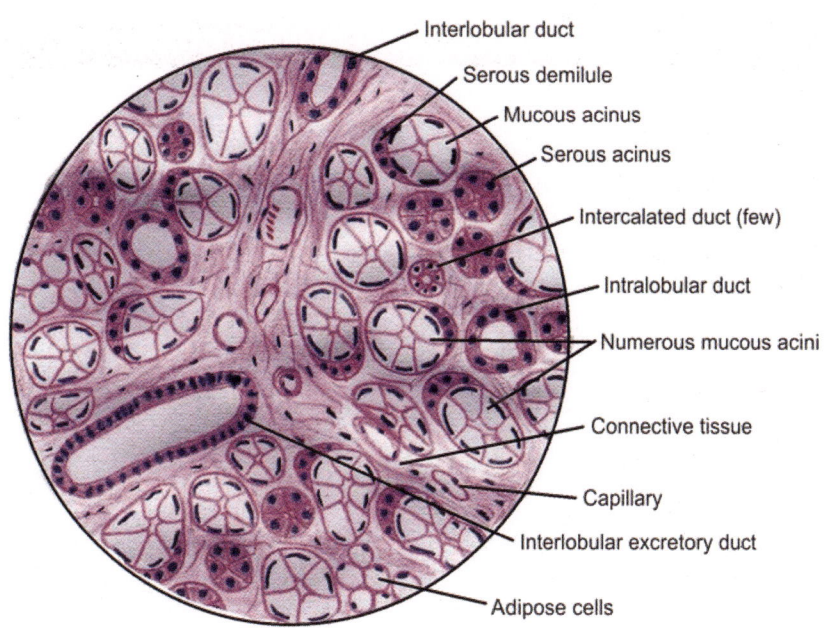

Interlobular duct
Serous demilule
Mucous acinus
Serous acinus
Intercalated duct (few)
Intralobular duct
Numerous mucous acini
Connective tissue
Capillary
Interlobular excretory duct
Adipose cells

Date:

PAROTID SALIVARY GLAND (SEROUS GLAND)

SPECIFIC LEARNING OBJECTIVES

At the end of the session the student should be able to:

1. Identify serous gland under light microscope.
2. Identify the serous acini, ducts, connective tissue.
3. Explain what serous secretion looks like in H & E stain and why.
4. Draw the microanatomy of serous salivary gland.

Distribution and function of serous glands

_____

_____

_____

_____

Three points of identification

_____

_____

_____

_____

_____

_____

Date:

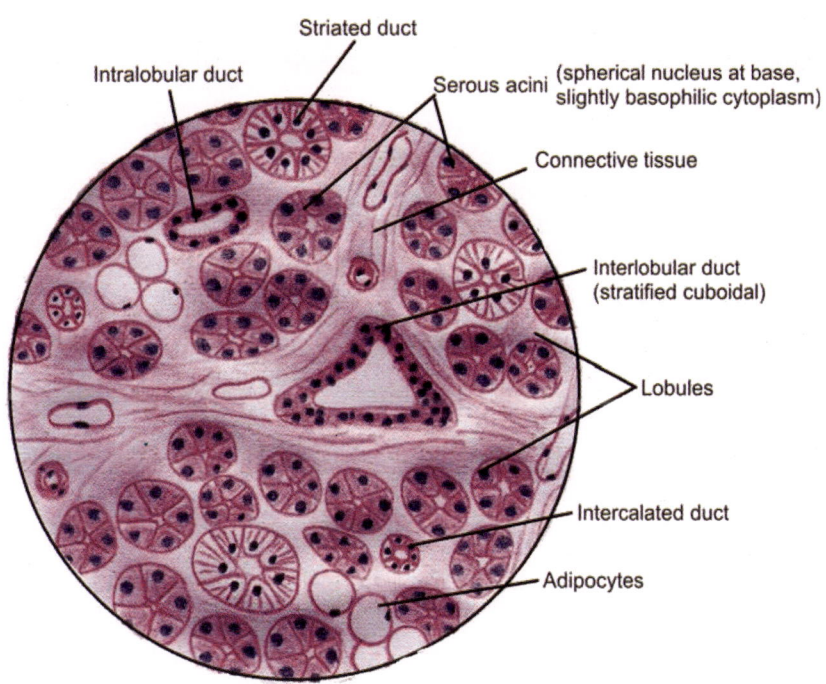

Striated duct

Intralobular duct

Serous acini (spherical nucleus at base, slightly basophilic cytoplasm)

Connective tissue

Interlobular duct (stratified cuboidal)

Lobules

Intercalated duct

Adipocytes

Date:

SUBMANDIBULAR SALIVARY GLAND (MIXED GLAND)

SPECIFIC LEARNING OBJECTIVES

At the end of the session the student should be able to:

1. Identify mixed salivary gland under light microscope.
2. Identify the mucous and serous acini, ducts, connective tissue.
3. Identify the serous demilunes.
4. Draw the microanatomy of mixed salivary gland.

Distribution and function of mixed glands

_____

_____

_____

_____

Three points of identification

_____

_____

_____

_____

_____

_____

Date:

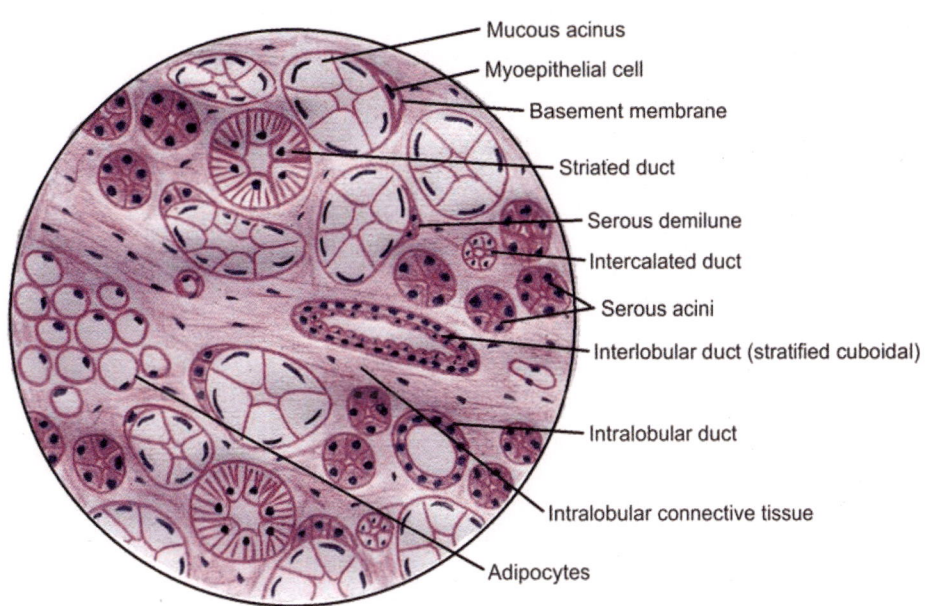

- Mucous acinus
- Myoepithelial cell
- Basement membrane
- Striated duct
- Serous demilune
- Intercalated duct
- Serous acini
- Interlobular duct (stratified cuboidal)
- Intralobular duct
- Intralobular connective tissue
- Adipocytes

Date:

SDL NOTES

Date:

SDL NOTES

Date:

BLOOD VESSELS HISTOLOGY

Number	Competency	Domain	Level	Core (Y/N)	Teaching/learning method	Assessment method	Number required to certify
AN 69.1	Identify elastic and muscular blood vessels, capillaries under the microscope	K/S	SH	Y	Lecture, practical	Written/skill assessment	
AN 69.2	Describe the various types and structure-function correlation of blood vessels	K	KH	Y	Lecture, practical	Written	
AN 69.3	Describe the ultrastructure of blood vessels	K	KH	Y	Lecture, practical	Written	

THINK AND ANSWER

1. Large arteries (like aorta, brachiocephalic trunk, common carotid, common iliac, etc.) receive lots of blood under pressure in each systole. Then the blood passes forwards and the wall of arteries recoil. So what kind of tissue should be present in the wall of large blood vessels?
2. You already know the epithelium lining of the lumen. What is it?
3. If a blood vessel can constrict or dilate then which tissue will be responsible for this?

Elastic Artery

- The diameter of the lumen is usually more than the thickness of the wall.
- It consists of 3 layers: Tunica intima, tunica media and tunica adventitia.
- Tunica intima has endothelium (of simple squamous epithelium), sub-endothelial connective tissue and internal elastic lamina. The internal elastic lamina is not well developed in elastic artery.
- Tunica media is the thickest layer and mainly has elastic fibres apart from few smooth muscle fibres.
- Tunica adventitia has collagenous connective tissue fibres with vasa vasorum and autonomic nerves.

Muscular Arteries

- The diameter of the lumen is usually less than the thickness of the wall. Layers are the same as elastic artery. The difference is that the tunica intima shows folding due to the prominent internal elastic lamina which is wavy, formed of condensed elastic fibres.
- The tunica media has concentrically arranged smooth muscle fibres. Very few elastic fibres are present.

Vein

- Wall of veins is thin and lumen is collapsed. Small and medium sized veins have valves.
- The 3 layers are the same with the following differences:
  o Internal elastic lamina is absent in tunica intima.
  o Tunica media is thin and has very few elastic tissue and muscle fibres.
  o Tunica adventitia is well developed and thicker than the tunica media. It has collagen fibres, smooth muscle fibres, and few elastic fibres.

Capillaries

- The wall of capillary is formed of a single layer of endothelial cells and basal lamina. Occasionally a pericyte may be seen outside the basal lamina of continuous capillaries. Pericyte is a contractile cell.

Date:

Ultrastructure of Capillaries

Capillaries are of 3 types:

1. Continuous capillary—here there are no fenestrations in the endothelial cells or basal lamina, e.g. capillaries of muscles, nervous tissue, etc.
2. Fenestrated capillary—fenestrations of 70–90 micrometer diameter are present in the endothelium, through which passage of fluid or blood components occurs. Basal lamina is continuous, e.g. capillaries of small intestine, glomeruli, endocrine glands, etc.
3. Sinusoidal capillaries—these are large and irregular in shape. Endothelium is fenestrated and basal lamina is also not continuous, e.g. capillaries of liver, spleen, bone marrow.

Draw the Microanatomy of the Given Capillary and Vein with Proper H & E Staining and Labelling

CAPILLARY Draw a capillary according to the description given above	VEIN

Date:

ELASTIC ARTERY/ LARGE ARTERY

SPECIFIC LEARNING OBJECTIVES

At the end of the session the student should be able to:

1. Identify elastic artery under light microscope.
2. Identify the 3 layers of blood vessels.
3. Identify the elastic fibres in tunica media.
4. Draw a diagram of microanatomy of elastic artery.

Distribution and function

_____

_____

_____

_____

Three points of identification

_____

_____

_____

_____

_____

_____

Date:

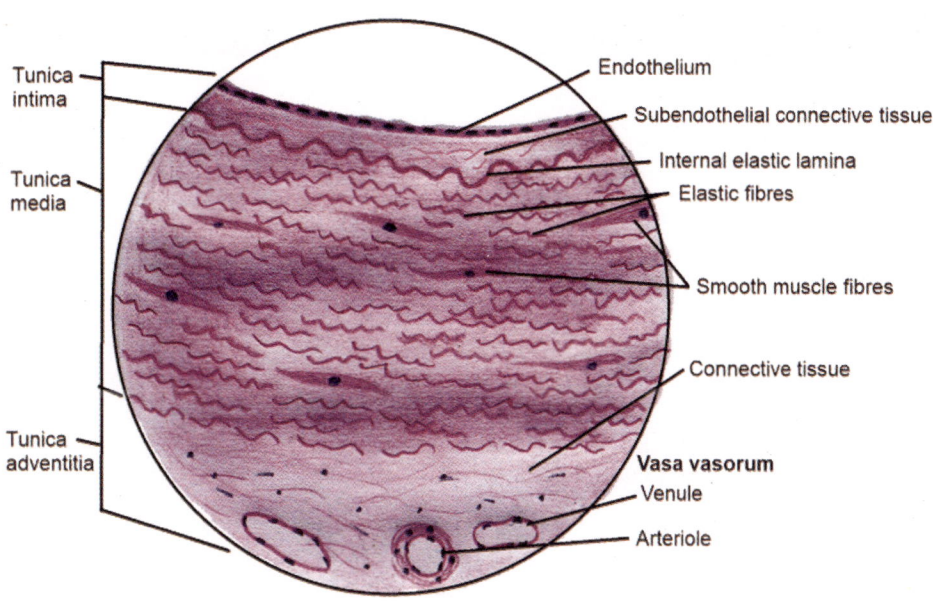

Tunica intima

Tunica media

Tunica adventitia

Endothelium

Subendothelial connective tissue

Internal elastic lamina

Elastic fibres

Smooth muscle fibres

Connective tissue

Vasa vasorum

Venule

Arteriole

Date:

MUSCULAR ARTERY/MEDIUM SIZED ARTERY

SPECIFIC LEARNING OBJECTIVES

At the end of the session the student should be able to:

1. Identify muscular artery under light microscope.
2. Identify the 3 layers of blood vessels.
3. Identify the internal elastic lamina
4. Identify the muscle fibres in tunica media.
5. Identify external elastic lamina.
6. Draw a diagram of microanatomy of muscular artery.

Distribution and correlation of structure with function of muscular artery

_____

_____

_____

_____

Three points of identification

_____

_____

_____

_____

_____

_____

Date:

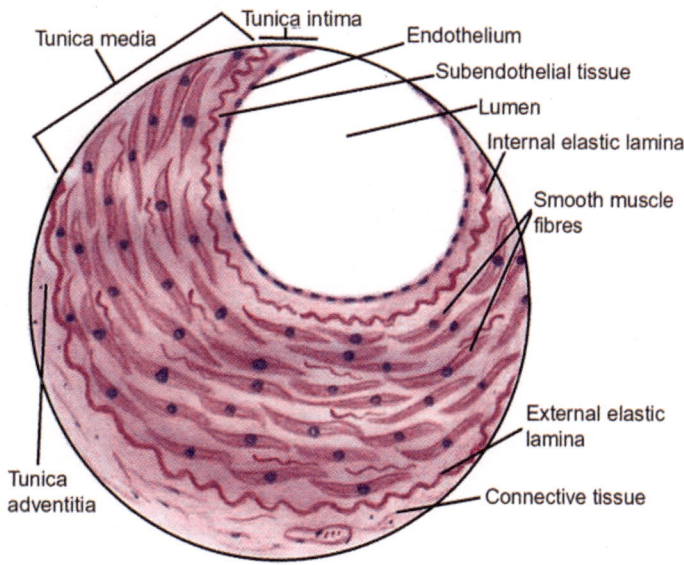

Date:

SDL NOTES

Date:

SDL NOTES

Date:

LYMPHOID TISSUE

Number	Competency	Domain	Level	Core (Y/N)	Teaching/learning method	Assessment method	Number required to certify
AN70.2	Identify the lymphoid tissue under the microscope and describe microanatomy of lymph node, spleen, thymus, tonsil and correlate the structure with function	K/S	SH	Y	Lecture, practical	Written/skill assessment	

Dense lymphoid tissue is an aggregation of lymphocytes which are arranged in the form of nodules. Therefore the microscopic appearance is similar to lymphocytes in H & E stain apart from the connective tissue within and outside the tissue and its blood vessels. The scope of this book deals with structures mentioned in the competencies above.

Think and Answer

1. What will be the colour taken up by the predominant cells (lymphocytes) in lymphoid tissue if stained by H & E?

_____

_____

2. What will be the colour of connective tissue fibres within the tissue?

_____

_____

3. What is the function of spleen? So what do you expect to see in its microanatomy?

_____

_____

_____

4. What is the function of thymus? So what kind of cells do you expect to see under the light microscope?

_____

_____

_____

5. Does the thymus persist till adulthood? If not, then do you expect to see some degenerative changes under the light microscope?

_____

_____

_____

6. Where are palatine tonsils situated? So what kind of epithelium should be present on the side facing the oral cavity?

_____

Date:

LYMPH NODE

- It has an outer zone of densely packed lymphocytes in the form of aggregates called lymphoid follicles or lymphoid nodules. The nodule has a densely packed dark (basophilic) stained peripheral region and a paler staining germinal centre.
- The central zone, medulla, is light stained with lymphocytes arranged as cords.
- Lymph node is surrounded by a capsule made up of mainly collagen fibres. The capsule sends septae (trabeculae) within the node to divide into lobules.
- There is subcapsular sinus just below the capsule. It contains lymph which enters the LN through convex side of LN. Then this lymph flows through the sinuses present along the trabeculae called cortical sinuses. This reaches the medulla where there are medullary sinuses which join to form efferent lymphatic vessels which emerge through the hilum.
- Blood vessels enter the hilum and pass through the medulla to reach the cortex.

Now Answeer these Questions

1. What stain will lymph take on H & E staining?

_____

_____

_____

2. So what will be the colour of sinuses?

_____

_____

_____

3. What is the characteristic of lining epithelium of sinuses?

_____

_____

_____

4. Where do you expect to see the blood vessels in lymph node?

_____

_____

_____

Date:

SPECIFIC LEARNING OBJECTIVES

At the end of the session the student should be able to:
1. Identify lymph node under light microscope.
2. Identify the lymphatic follicles, cortex and medulla.
3. Identify the subcapsular and medullary sinuses.
4. Identify the capsule and trabeculae.
5. Draw the microanatomy of lymph node.

Distribution and function

_____

_____

_____

_____

Three points of identification

_____

_____

_____

_____

_____

_____

Date:

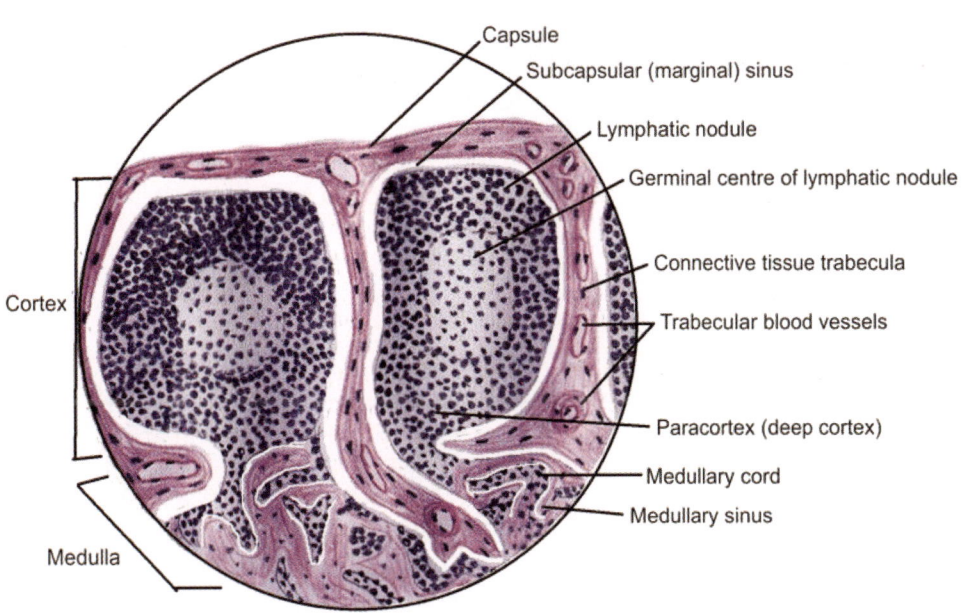

- Capsule
- Subcapsular (marginal) sinus
- Lymphatic nodule
- Germinal centre of lymphatic nodule
- Connective tissue trabecula
- Trabecular blood vessels
- Paracortex (deep cortex)
- Medullary cord
- Medullary sinus

Cortex

Medulla

Date:

SPLEEN

- Outermost is a layer of mesothelium (can you tell what kind of epithelium is present in mesothelium? _____). Spleen is surrounded by dense connective tissue-capsule. It sends trabeculae inside the substance of spleen. Blood vessels enter along the trabeculae.
- The arrangement of lymphoid tissue in spleen is not like cortex and medulla. Instead it is arranged as red pulp and white pulp.
- The characteristic reticular fibre network of spleen is not visible in H & E staining.

WHITE PULP

- The arteries enter the parenchyma as arterioles and are surrounded by a sheath of T lymphocytes. This sheath is known as periarterial lymphatic sheath (PALS). So these will appear as cords because the arteriole extends in length and it is surrounded by PALS. If cut in TS it appears round with central artery.
- At places the arrangement of lymphocytes becomes nodular and these are known as lymphatic nodules. These nodules have B lymphocytes with a light stained and loosely packed germinal centre surrounded by densely packed dark staining peripheral lymphocytes. These nodules are known as malpighian bodies.
- There is a central arteriole which is eccentric in position. This arteriole usually lies between the germinal centre and densely packed lymphocytes. This is the characteristic and differentiating feature of lymphatic nodule of spleen.

RED PULP

- This is another characteristic feature of microscopic structure of spleen. The red pulp consists of all cells of blood. There are sinusoids (can you tell the lining epithelium of sinusoids? _____) which are surrounded by cords of blood cells (T lymphocytes, B lymphocytes, macrophages, other cells of blood). These cords are known as cords of Billroth. The red pulp surrounding the lymphatic nodule is made of sinusoids and is known as marginal zone.

SPLENIC CIRCULATION

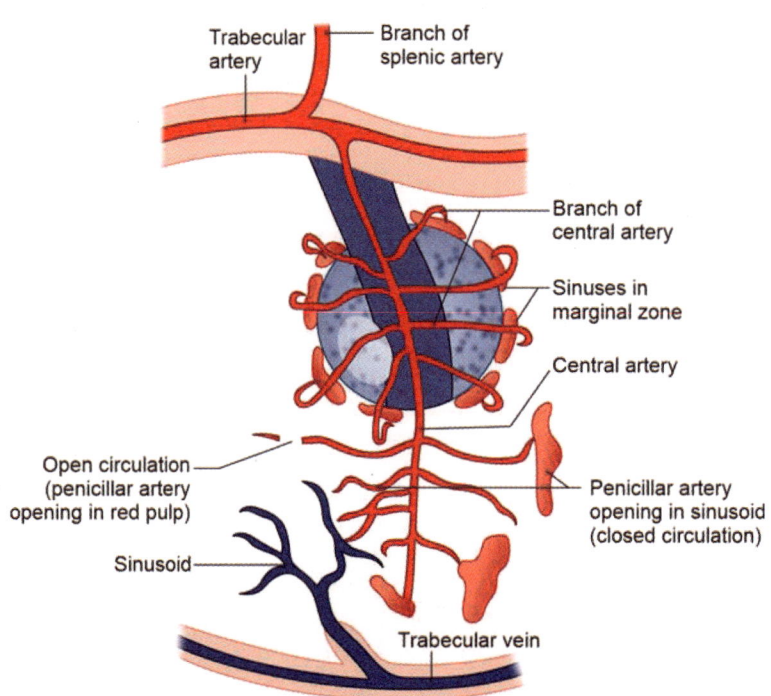

Date:

SPECIFIC LEARNING OBJECTIVES

At the end of the session the student should be able to:

1. Identify spleen under light microscope.
2. Identify red pulp and white pulp.
3. Identify central artery in white pulp.
4. Identify medullary cords and sinuses.
5. Draw a diagram of microanatomy of spleen.

Function of red and white pulps

_____

_____

_____

_____

Three points of identification

_____

_____

_____

_____

_____

_____

Date:

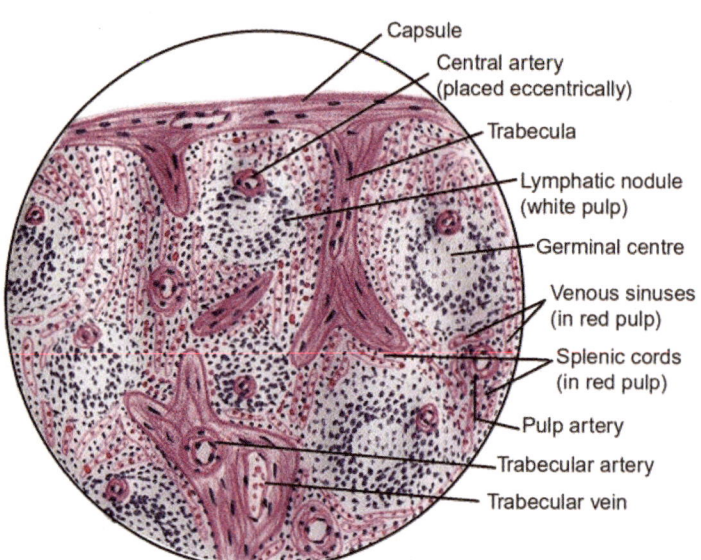

- Capsule
- Central artery (placed eccentrically)
- Trabecula
- Lymphatic nodule (white pulp)
- Germinal centre
- Venous sinuses (in red pulp)
- Splenic cords (in red pulp)
- Pulp artery
- Trabecular artery
- Trabecular vein

Date:

THYMUS

- Thymus is divided into incomplete lobules by septae from capsule.
- Thus there is cortex in the periphery and medulla in the centre of each lobule.
- Medulla is placed in the centre and communicates with the medulla of adjoining incomplete lobules.
- Cortex of thymus contains densely packed T lymphocytes, epithelioreticular cells (epitheliocytes) and macrophages.
- Medulla contains fewer lymphocytes but more epitheliocytes. Concentrically arranged degenerating epitheliocytes form Hassall's corpuscles or thymic corpuscles (characteristic feature of thymus).
- Composition of Hassall's corpuscles: Degenerating epitheliocytes, lipid and macrophages.

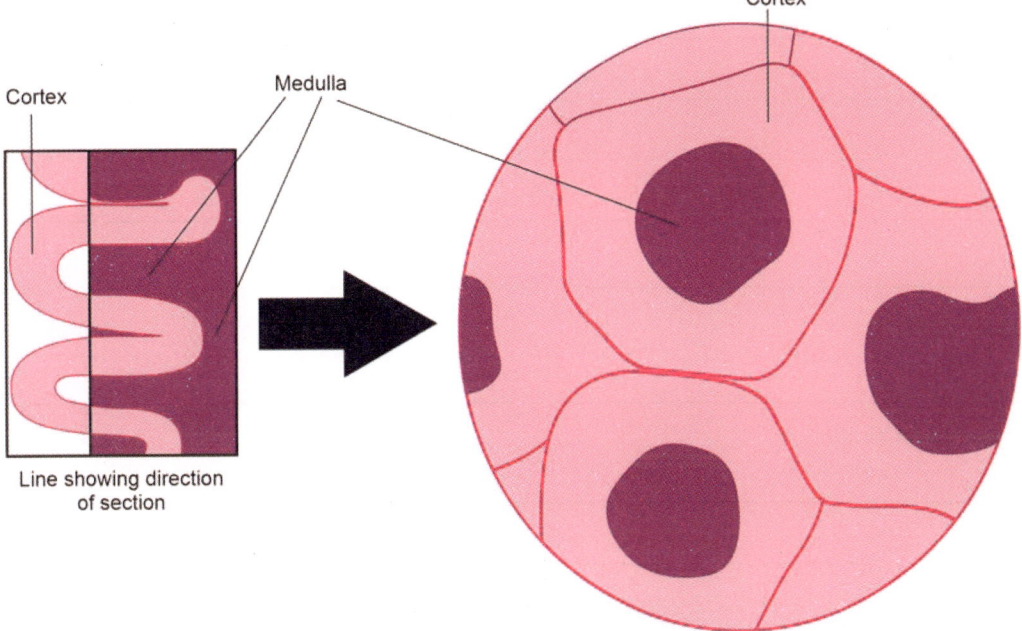

Cortex

Medulla

Cortex

Line showing direction of section

Answer the Following

1. What are Hassall's corpuscles?

_____

_____

_____

_____

2. What are the changes in thymus gland with advancing age?

_____

_____

_____

_____

_____

Date:

SPECIFIC LEARNING OBJECTIVES

At the end of the session the student should be able to:

1. Identify thymus under the light microscope.
2. Identify its lobules and cortex and medulla.
3. Identify the lymphoid cells.
4. Identify Hassall's corpuscles.
5. Draw a diagram of microanatomy of thymus.

Distribution and Function of thymus

_____

_____

_____

_____

Three points of identification

_____

_____

_____

_____

_____

_____

Date:

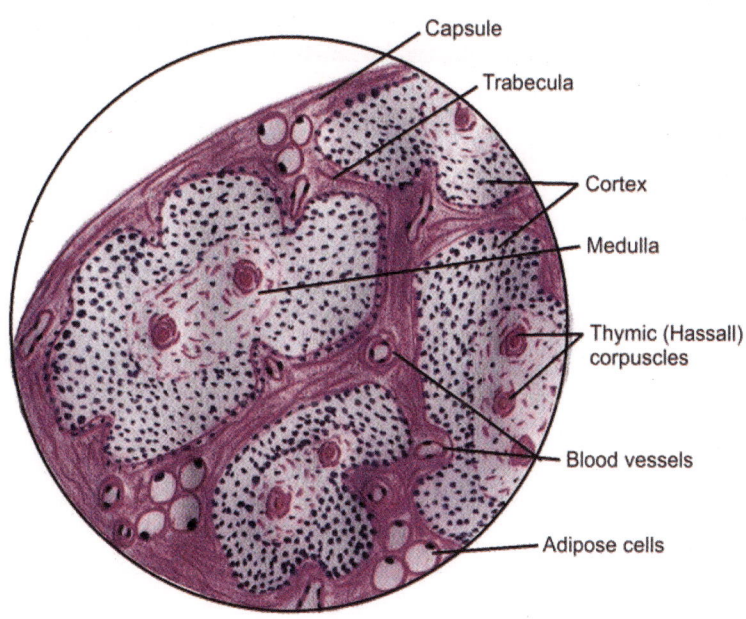

Capsule

Trabecula

Cortex

Medulla

Thymic (Hassall) corpuscles

Blood vessels

Adipose cells

Date:

PALATINE TONSIL

- Tonsils are collections of lymphoid tissues.
- Palatine tonsil is present in the junction of oral cavity with pharynx. As such the covering epithelium is same as that of the oral cavity, i.e. stratified squamous non-keratinized.
- Tonsillar crypts are seen as extensions of covering epithelium within the substance of the tonsil.

Revise and Answer

1. What are the features of stratified squamous non-keratinized epithelium?

_____

_____

_____

_____

2. How can you correlate tonsillar crypts with development of palatine tonsils?

_____

_____

_____

_____

_____

_____

3. What kind of muscles fibres (smooth/skeletal) may be seen on the deeper side of palatine tonsils?

_____

_____

_____

_____

_____

4. Name the other tonsils participating in the formation of Waldeyer's ring.

_____

_____

_____

_____

_____

_____

Date:

SPECIFIC LEARNING OBJECTIVES

At the end of the session the student should be able to:

1. Identify palatine tonsil under the light microscope.
2. Identify lymphoid nodules in the tissue.
3. Identify stratified squamous epithelial lining of the tissue.
4. Identify tonsillar crypts.
5. Identify muscle fibres in the deeper side of palatine tonsil (if present in section).
6. Draw a diagram of microanatomy of palatine tonsil.

Function of lymphoid nodules

_____

_____

_____

_____

Three points of identification

_____

_____

_____

_____

_____

_____

Date:

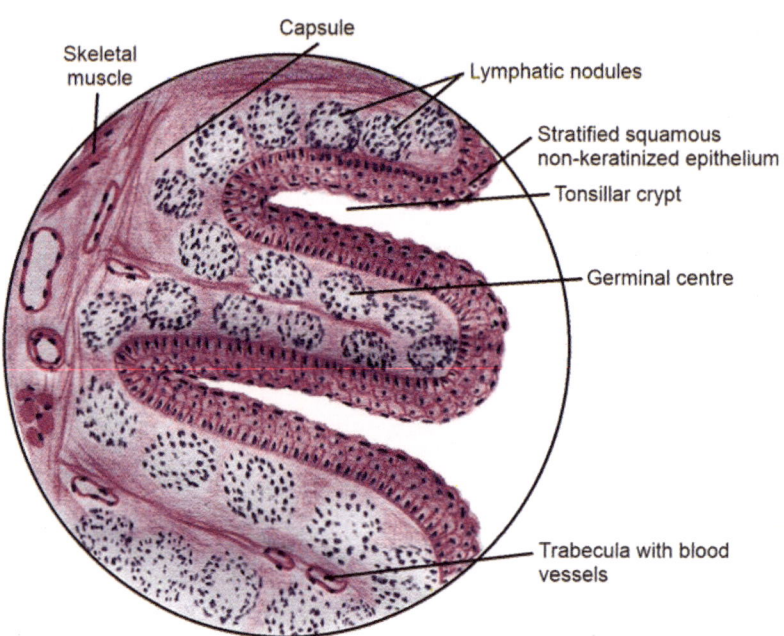

- Skeletal muscle
- Capsule
- Lymphatic nodules
- Stratified squamous non-keratinized epithelium
- Tonsillar crypt
- Germinal centre
- Trabecula with blood vessels

Date:

SDL NOTES

Date:

SDL NOTES

Date:

INTEGUMENTARY SYSTEM

Number	Competency	Domain	Level	Core (Y/N)	Teaching/learning method	Assessment method	Number required to certify
AN 72.1	Identify the skin and its appendages under the microscope and correlate the structure with function	K/S	SH	Y	Lecture, practical	Written/skill assessment	

The skin consists of epidermis and dermis. Epidermis is made up of five layers:

1. Stratum basale—deepest layer of columnar or cuboidal cells
2. Stratum spinosum—polygonal cells.
3. Stratum granulosum—2–5 flat cell layers.
4. Stratum lucidum—appears clear and the cell boundaries are not well defined. This layer is absent or inconspicuous in thin skin.
5. Stratum corneum—most superficial layer. There are no cells, only scaly elements in keratin are present. (What is the appearance of keratin in H & E stain?)

Appendages of Skin

1. Hair—it has a shaft and a root. Hair follicle is lined by cells derived from the layers of skin. It is found in thin skin.
2. Arrector pili muscles—smooth muscles in dermis which contract on stimulation and make the hair to stand on end.
3. Sebaceous glands—holocrine glands in dermis associated with hair follicles. Alveoli of glands can be seen. The tarsal glands (Meibomian glands) of eyelid are modified sebaceous glands.
4. Sweat glands present in the dermis. Secretory part of the gland is made up of cuboidal or low columnar cells. Its duct is lined by stratified cuboidal epithelium. They are more numerous in thick skin.
5. Nails

Date:

THIN SKIN

SPECIFIC LEARNING OBJECTIVES

At the end of the session the student should be able to:

1. Identify thin skin under the light microscope.
2. Identify epidermis and dermis of skin
3. Identify hair follicles
4. Identify sebaceous glands, sweat glands and sweat ducts
5. Identify arrector pili muscles.
6. Draw a diagram of microanatomy of thin skin.

Distribution and function

_____

_____

_____

_____

Three points of identification

_____

_____

_____

_____

_____

_____

Date:

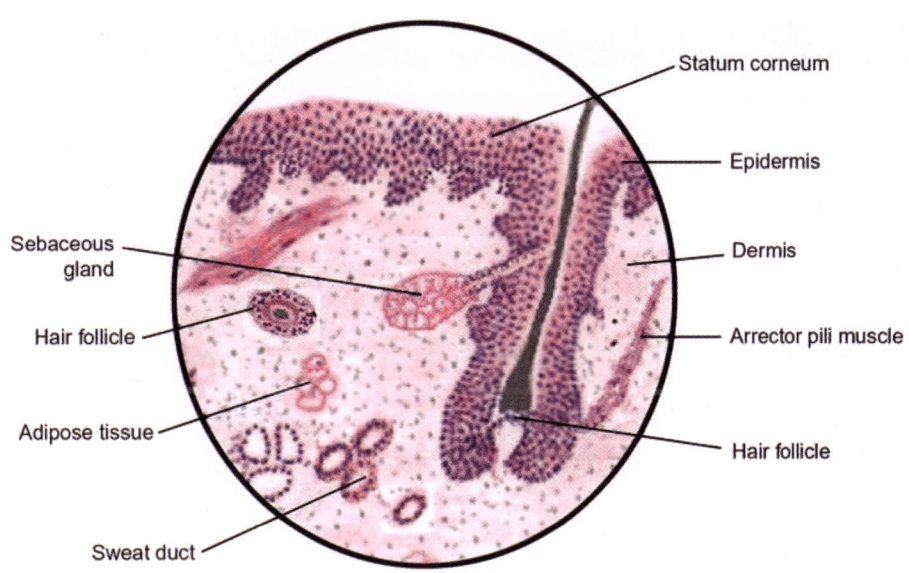

Statum corneum

Epidermis

Dermis

Arrector pili muscle

Hair follicle

Sebaceous gland

Hair follicle

Adipose tissue

Sweat duct

Date:

THICK SKIN

SPECIFIC LEARNING OBJECTIVES

At the end of the session the student should be able to:
1. Identify thick skin under the light microscope
2. Identify absence of hair follicles.
3. Identify the dermis and epidermis.
4. Identify the kind of epithelium with keratinisation.
5. Identify the adipocytes, sweat glands.
6. Draw a diagram of microanatomy of thick skin.

Distribution and function

_____

_____

_____

_____

Three points of identification

_____

_____

_____

_____

_____

_____

Date:

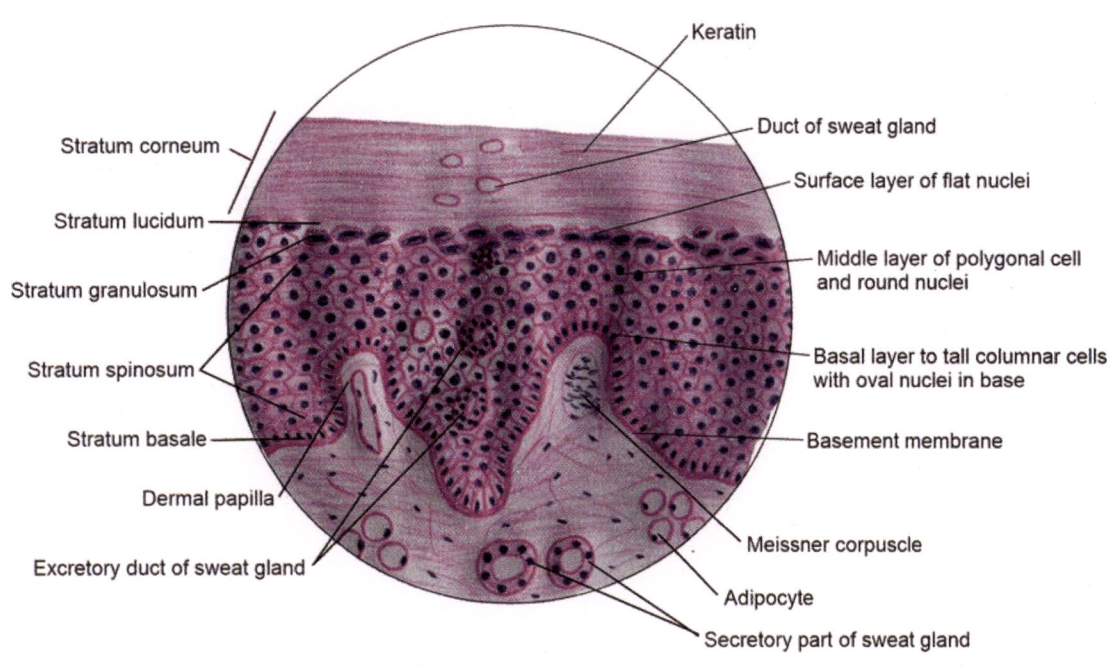

- Keratin
- Duct of sweat gland
- Surface layer of flat nuclei
- Middle layer of polygonal cell and round nuclei
- Basal layer to tall columnar cells with oval nuclei in base
- Basement membrane
- Meissner corpuscle
- Adipocyte
- Secretory part of sweat gland

- Stratum corneum
- Stratum lucidum
- Stratum granulosum
- Stratum spinosum
- Stratum basale
- Dermal papilla
- Excretory duct of sweat gland

Date:

SDL NOTES

Date:

SDL NOTES

Date:

RESPIRATORY SYSTEM						
Number	Competency	Domain	Level	Core (Y/N)	Teaching/learning method	Assessment method	Number required to certify
AN 25.1	Identify, draw and label a slide of trachea and lung	K/S	SH	Y	Lecture, practical	Written/skill assessment	1

TRACHEA

- It has pseudostratified ciliated columnar epithelium with goblet cells resting on a basement membrane.
- Lamina propria has elastic fibres, WBCs and ducts of glands.
- Submucosa has both mucous and serous acini.
- C-shaped hyaline cartilage lies beneath the submucosa. The posterior gap in the cartilage has smooth muscle fibres known as trachealis.
- Adventitia is the outermost layer.

Answer the Following

1. What type of cartilage is present in the trachea? What is its shape?

_____

_____

2. Why does the lumen of trachea not collapse?

_____

_____

3. How are chondrocytes arranged in the cartilage—groups or single?

_____

_____

4. What is the outer lining of cartilage known as?

_____

_____

5. What is the appearance of ground substance of hyaline cartilage in H & E stain and why?

_____

_____

_____

6. What kind of epithelium lining do you expect for trapping foreign particles in the inspired air?

_____

_____

7. What is the lining epithelium of trachea?

_____

_____

8. What is the nature of secretion by glands in trachea?

_____

_____

Date:

TRACHEA

SPECIFIC LEARNING OBJECTIVES

At the end of the session the student should be able to:

1. Identify trachea under the light microscope.
2. Identify the pseudostratified ciliated columnar epithelium with goblet cells.
3. Identify the hyaline cartilage, perichondrium, chondrocytes, lacunae and homogenous ground substance.
4. Identify the mucous and serous glands between cartilage and epithelium
5. Identify smooth muscle—trachealis
6. Draw a diagram of microanatomy of trachea.

Distribution and function of pseudostratified epithelium

_____

_____

_____

_____

Three points of identification

_____

_____

_____

_____

_____

_____

Date:

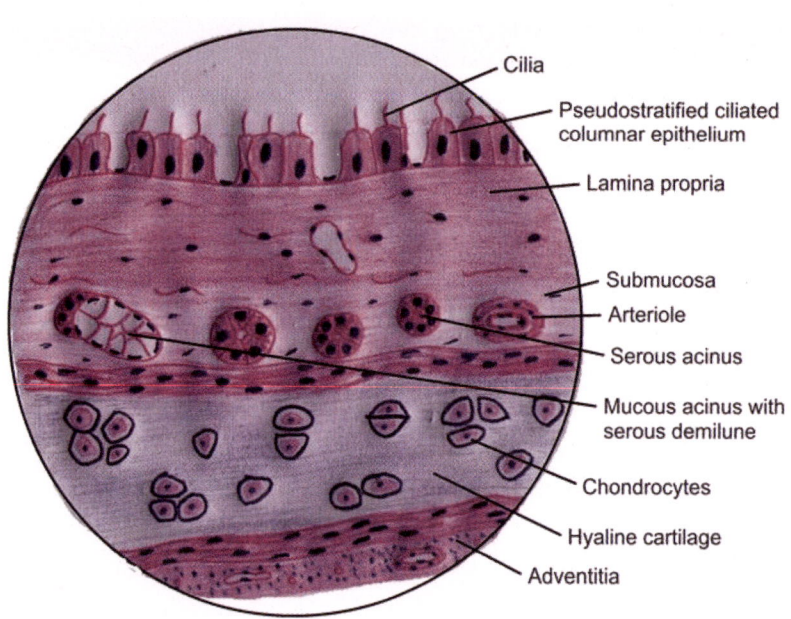

- Cilia
- Pseudostratified ciliated columnar epithelium
- Lamina propria
- Submucosa
- Arteriole
- Serous acinus
- Mucous acinus with serous demilune
- Chondrocytes
- Hyaline cartilage
- Adventitia

Date:

LUNG

- The surface of lung is covered by pleura (mesothelium).
- Lungs have airways which form the parenchyma and connective tissue which form the stroma.
- So the airway has principal bronchus, primary and secondary bronchi, bronchioles, terminal bronchioles and respiratory bronchioles; alveolar ducts, alveolar sacs and alveoli.
- Interalveolar septum is present between the adjacent alveoli. So there is connective tissue between the walls of adjacent alveoli. It also has collagen and elastic fibres and fibroblasts and macrophages.
- Capillaries in contact with alveolar walls help in gaseous exchange. Here the basement membrane of capillaries and alveoli fuse.
- When a section of lung is taken for H & E staining, it may show all the above structures or some may not be seen as they do not come in the section (e.g. principal bronchus may not be there in the section).
- Mucosa consists of epithelial lining and lamina propria.
- The epithelial lining and cartilage of each of the structures mentioned above is as follows:

Part	Lining epithelium	Cartilage
Intrapulmonary bronchus	Pseudostratified ciliated columnar epithelium with goblet cells	Plates of hyaline cartilage present (not C-shaped) up to tertiary bronchi
Bronchiole	Simple ciliated columnar in larger bronchioles and non-ciliated in smaller bronchioles	Absent
Terminal bronchiole (diameter <1 mm)	Simple non-ciliated columnar, no goblet cells. Dome shaped clara cells are present.	Absent
Respiratory bronchiole	Cuboidal epithelium. Simple squamous near opening of alveoli	Absent
Alveolar duct	Simple squamous epithelium	—
Alveolar sac	Simple squamous epithelium	—
Alveoli	Single layer of cells—type I, and type II pneumocytes—cuboidal cells (lesser in number)	

- Under the lamina propria there are smooth muscle fibres distal to trachea.
- Submucosa has mucous and serous glands in the proximal airways up to the level of tertiary bronchii.
- The alveoli give a honey comb appearance under a light microscope.

Date:

SPECIFIC LEARNING OBJECTIVES

At the end of the session the student should be able to:

1. Identify lung under the light microscope.
2. Identify honey-comb appearing alveoli lined by simple squamous epithelium.
3. Identify intrapulmonary bronchi—pseudostratified ciliated columnar epithelium, hyaline cartilage
4. Identify respiratory bronchioles along with their smooth muscles.
5. Identify alveolar ducts and sacs.
6. Draw a diagram of microanatomy of lung.

Distribution and function of type II pneumocytes

_____

_____

_____

_____

Three points of identification

_____

_____

_____

_____

_____

_____

Date:

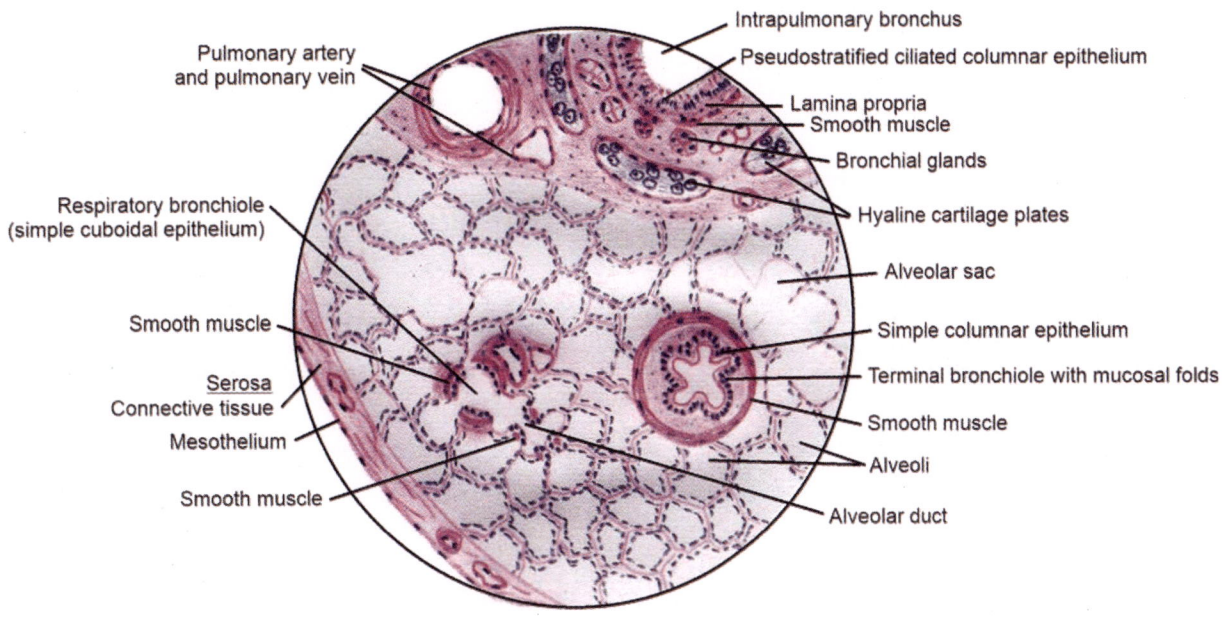

- Intrapulmonary bronchus
- Pseudostratified ciliated columnar epithelium
- Lamina propria
- Smooth muscle
- Bronchial glands
- Hyaline cartilage plates
- Alveolar sac
- Simple columnar epithelium
- Terminal bronchiole with mucosal folds
- Smooth muscle
- Alveoli
- Alveolar duct

- Pulmonary artery and pulmonary vein
- Respiratory bronchiole (simple cuboidal epithelium)
- Smooth muscle
- Serosa
- Connective tissue
- Mesothelium
- Smooth muscle

Date:

SDL NOTES

Date:

SDL NOTES

Date:

INTERALVEOLAR SEPTUM

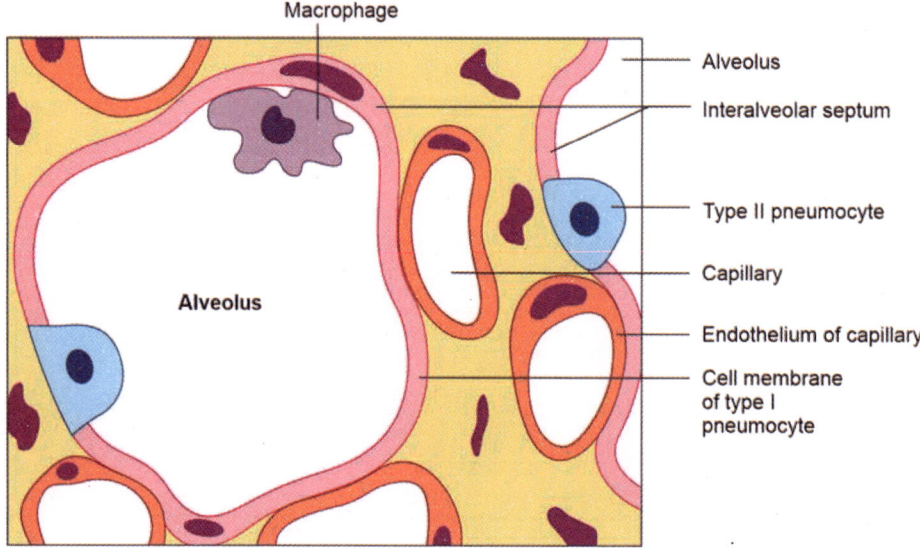

Macrophage

Alveolus

Alveolus

Interalveolar septum

Type II pneumocyte

Capillary

Endothelium of capillary

Cell membrane
of type I
pneumocyte

SPECIFIC LEARNING OBJECTIVES

At the end of the session the student should be able to:
1. Draw a diagram of microstructure of interalveolar septum.
2. Enumerate the type of cells present in alveoli and septum.
3. Write the functions of various cells.
4. Describe the blood-air barrier.

Interalveolar Septum

Date:

Answer the Following

1. Enumerate the cells present in alveoli and interalveolar septum.

_____

_____

_____

_____

_____

2. Write the functions of type I and type II pneumocytes.

_____

_____

_____

_____

_____

_____

3. Write the layers of blood–air barrier.

_____

_____

_____

_____

_____

_____

Date:

EPIGLOTTIS

- As evident from the given diagram, epiglottis has two surfaces: One facing the oral side and the other facing the respiratory passage.
- There is elastic cartilage in the epiglottis.

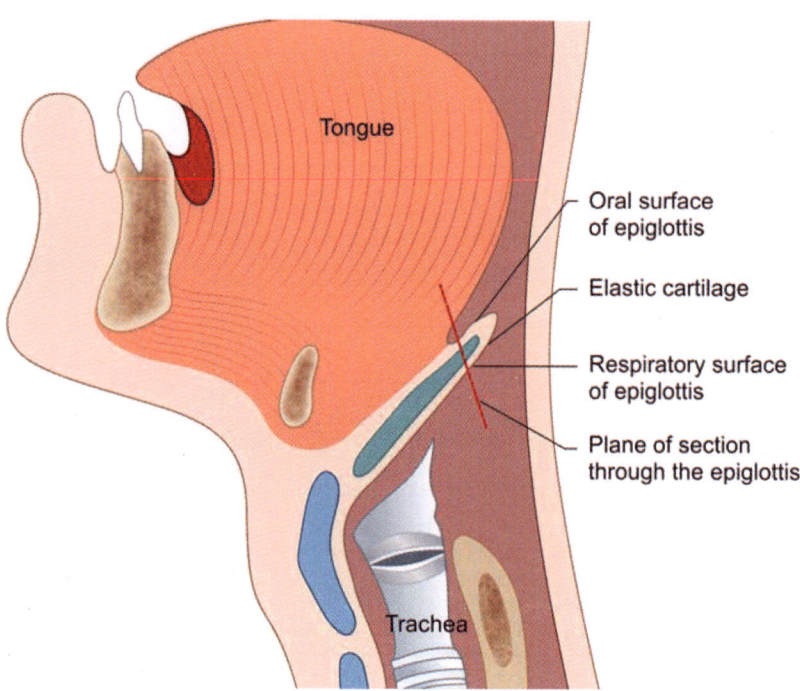

Think and Answer

1. What is the epithelial lining of the oral side of epiglottis?

_____

_____

_____

2. What is the epithelial lining of the side of epiglottis facing the respiratory passage?

_____

_____

_____

3. What are the microanatomical features of the cartilage of epiglottis?

_____

_____

_____

Layers of Epiglottis

- Stratified squamous epithelium
- Lamina propria having seromucinous glands.
- Elastic cartilage surrounded with perichondrium.
- Pseudostratified columnar epithelium with lamina propria and seromucinous glands.

Date:

SPECIFIC LEARNING OBJECTIVES

At the end of the session the student should be able to:

1. Identify epiglottis under the light microscope.
2. Identify stratified squamous non-keratinized epithelium.
3. Identify elastic cartilage.
4. Identify lamina propria and seromucinous glands within it.
5. Identify pseudostratified columnar epithelium.
6. Draw a diagram of microanatomy of epiglottis.

Distribution and function of elastic cartilage

_____

_____

_____

_____

Three points of identification

_____

_____

_____

_____

_____

_____

Date:

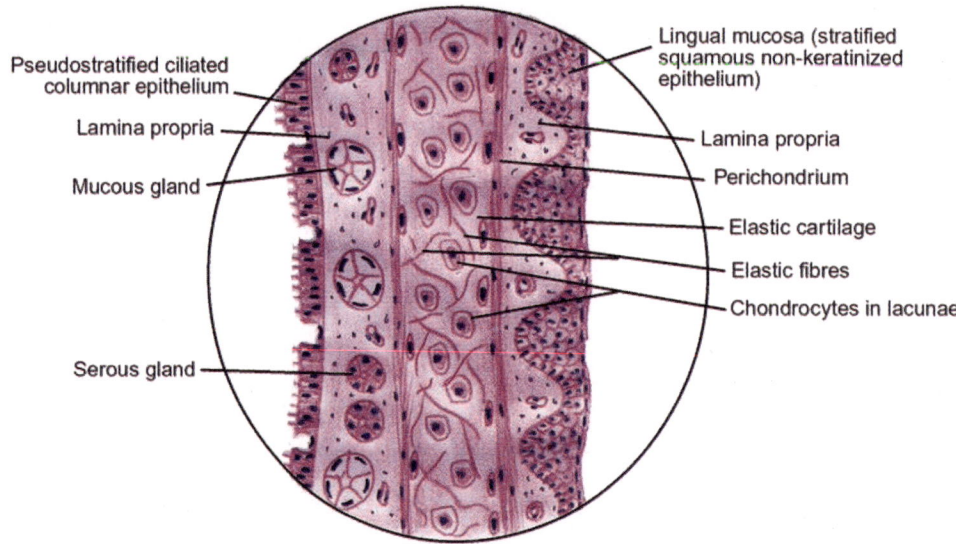

Pseudostratified ciliated columnar epithelium

Lamina propria

Mucous gland

Serous gland

Lingual mucosa (stratified squamous non-keratinized epithelium)

Lamina propria

Perichondrium

Elastic cartilage

Elastic fibres

Chondrocytes in lacunae

Date:

SDL NOTES

Date:

SDL NOTES

Date:

GASTROINTESTINAL SYSTEM

Number	Competency	Domain	Level	Core (Y/N)	Teaching/learning method	Assessment method	Number required to certify
AN 52.1	Describe and identify the microanatomical features of Gastrointestinal system: Oesophagus, fundus of stomach, pylorus of stomach, duodenum, jejunum, ileum, large intestine, appendix, liver, gall bladder, pancreas and suprarenals gland	K/S	SH	Y	Lecture, practical	Written/skill assessment	

General Layout of GIT

- There are four layers: Mucosa, submucosa, muscularis externa, serosa or adventitia.
- Mucosa is the lining epithelium along with lamina propria and muscularis interna. Lamina propria is connective tissue with blood supply, lymphatics, glands and lymphoid follicles.
- Submucosa consists of loose connective tissue. It may have glands also.
- Muscularis externa has two layers of smooth muscles—inner circular and outer longitudinal.
- Adventitia is loose connective tissue which is covered with mesothelium in the abdomen.
- Adventitia + mesothelium = Serosa.

Date:

TONGUE

Number	Competency	Domain	Level	Core (Y/N)	Teaching/learning method	Assessment method	Number required to certify
AN 43.2	Identify, describe and draw draw the microanatomy of pituitary gland, thyroid, parathyroid gland, tongue, salivary glands, tonsil, epiglottis, cornea, retina	K/S	SH	Y	Lecture, practical	Written/skill assessment	

Think and Answer

1. Can you move the tongue at your will? So what kind of muscle will be found in the tongue?

_____

_____

2. What is the special sense perceived by the tongue? So what will be found in histology?

_____

_____

3. What is the epithelial lining of oral cavity? Why?

_____

_____

- The oral cavity is lined by stratified squamous epithelium which is non-keratinized in most places. In the tongue the filiform papillae show keratinisation due to frequent mechanical stress.
- There is lamina propria but submucosa is absent in tongue. Lamina propria has minor salivary glands which are serous and mucous glands.
- The skeletal muscles of tongue run in different directions. So on section the fibres can be seen in different directions and sections as bundles.
- Taste buds are seen on circumvallate and fungiform papillae of tongue. Taste buds have oval cells arranged in clusters. At the apex of the taste bud there is a taste pore. The portion of cells towards the taste pore has microvilli.

Date:

SPECIFIC LEARNING OBJECTIVES

At the end of the session the student should be able to:

1. Identify tongue under the light microscope.
2. Identify its epithelium (stratified squamous non-keratinized).
3. Identify its papillae and taste buds.
4. Identify its skeletal muscles running in different directions.
5. Identify minor salivary glands.
6. Draw a diagram of microanatomy of tongue.

Distribution and function of taste buds and filiform papillae

_____

_____

_____

_____

Three points of identification

_____

_____

_____

_____

_____

_____

Date:

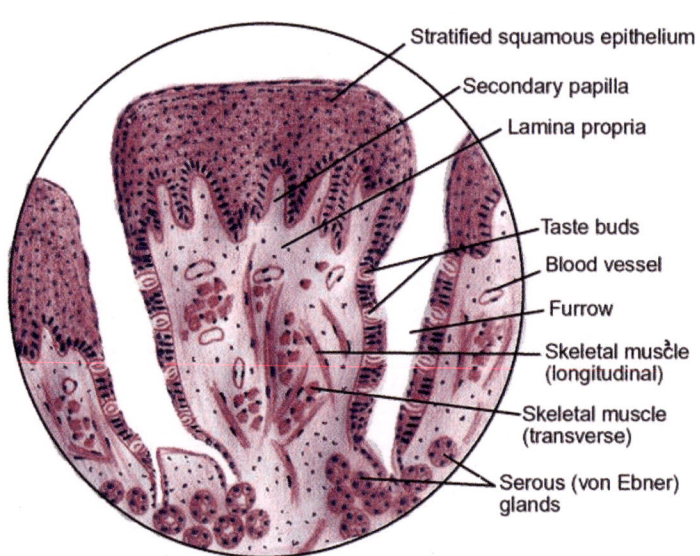

- Stratified squamous epithelium
- Secondary papilla
- Lamina propria
- Taste buds
- Blood vessel
- Furrow
- Skeletal muscle (longitudinal)
- Skeletal muscle (transverse)
- Serous (von Ebner) glands

Date:

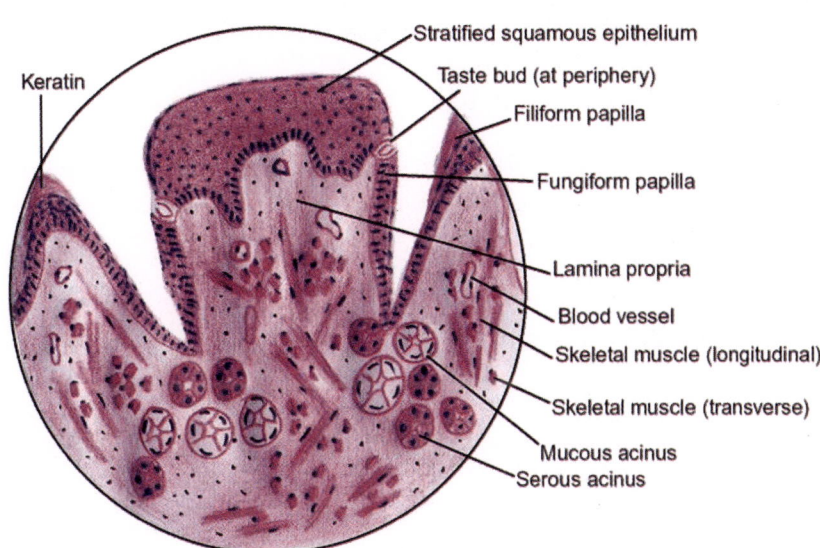

Keratin

Stratified squamous epithelium

Taste bud (at periphery)

Filiform papilla

Fungiform papilla

Lamina propria

Blood vessel

Skeletal muscle (longitudinal)

Skeletal muscle (transverse)

Mucous acinus

Serous acinus

Date:

OESOPHAGUS

The four layers are the same as the general plan of GIT.

1. Mucosa has stratified squamous non-keratinized epithelium. Lamina propria may have lymphoid follicles. Muscularis interna has smooth muscles.
2. Submucosa has mucous glands, blood vessels, lymphatics and Meissener's plexus of nerves.
3. Muscularis externa in the upper 1/3rd of oesophagus there are skeletal muscles, in middle 1/3rd there are smooth and skeletal muscles and lower 1/3rd there are only smooth muscles.
4. Outermost layer consists of adventitia in the upper part of oesophagus and serosa in abdominal part.

Think and Answer

a. Where all have you studied stratified squamous non-keratinized epithelium so far?

_____

_____

_____

_____

b. Smooth muscles are arranged circularly around the lumen. So if the oesophagus is cut transversely what will be the section through smooth muscles—transverse or longitudinal? How will it appear under the microscope?

_____

_____

_____

_____

_____

c. Similarly in muscularis externa what will be the section through inner circular layer if the gut is cut transversely? How will it appear under the microscope?

_____

_____

_____

_____

_____

d. What will be the section through outer longitudinal layer if the gut is cut transversely? How will it appear under the microscope?

_____

_____

_____

_____

_____

Date:

TS THROUGH LOWER ONE-THIRD OF OESOPHAGUS

SPECIFIC LEARNING OBJECTIVES

At the end of the session the student should be able to:

1. Identify oesophagus under the light microscope.
2. Identify the 4 layers of GIT.
3. Identify the stratified squamous non-keratinized epithelium of oesophagus.
4. Identify the oesophageal (mucous glands) in submucosa.
5. Identify the smooth muscle in muscularis externa.
6. Draw a diagram showing microanatomy of lower one-third of oesophagus.

Distribution of function of muscularis externa

_____

_____

_____

_____

Three points of identification

_____

_____

_____

_____

_____

_____

Date:

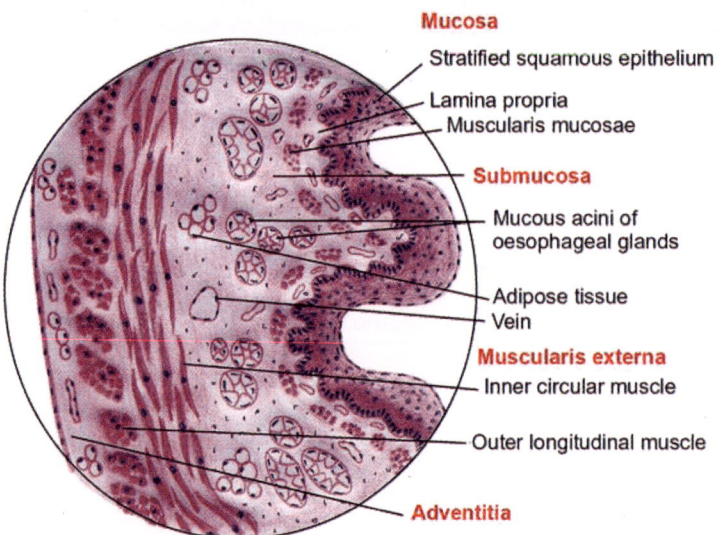

Mucosa

Stratified squamous epithelium

Lamina propria
Muscularis mucosae

Submucosa

Mucous acini of
oesophageal glands

Adipose tissue
Vein

Muscularis externa

Inner circular muscle

Outer longitudinal muscle

Adventitia

Date:

TS THROUGH UPPER ONE-THIRD OF OESOPHAGUS

SPECIFIC LEARNING OBJECTIVES

At the end of the session the student should be able to:

1. Identify oesophagus under the light microscope.
2. Identify the four layers of GIT.
3. Identify the stratified squamous non-keratinized epithelium of oesophagus.
4. Identify the oesophageal (mucous) glands in submucosa.
5. Identify the skeletal muscles in muscularis externa.
6. Draw a diagram of microanatomy of upper one-third of oesophagus.

Distribution of function of non-keratinized epithelium of oesophagus

_____

_____

_____

_____

Three points of identification

_____

_____

_____

_____

_____

_____

Date:

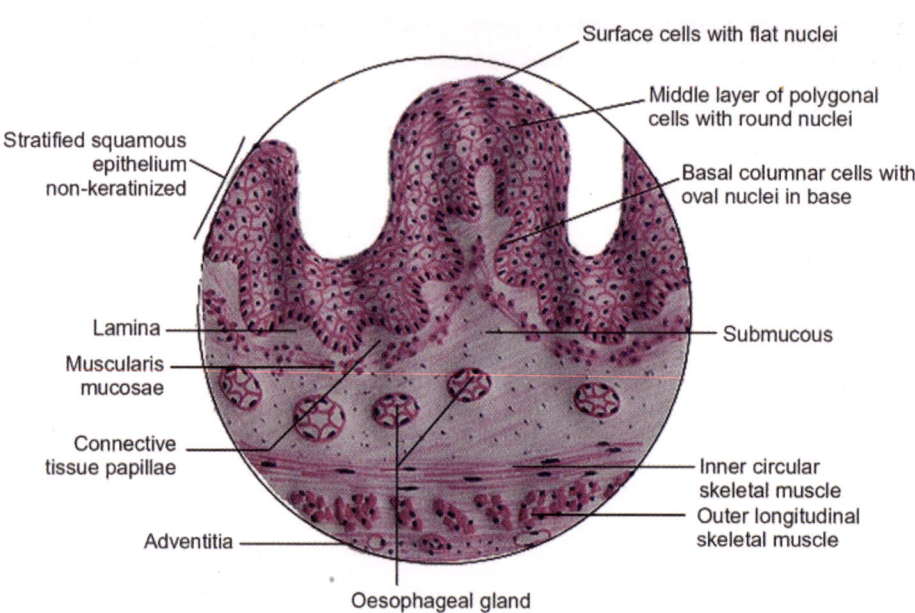

Surface cells with flat nuclei

Middle layer of polygonal cells with round nuclei

Basal columnar cells with oval nuclei in base

Stratified squamous epithelium non-keratinized

Lamina

Muscularis mucosae

Connective tissue papillae

Adventitia

Oesophageal gland

Submucous

Inner circular skeletal muscle

Outer longitudinal skeletal muscle

Date:

TS THROUGH MIDDLE ONE-THIRD OF OESOPHAGUS

SPECIFIC LEARNING OBJECTIVES

At the end of the session the student should be able to:

1. Identify oesophagus under the light microscope.
2. Identify the four layers of GIT.
3. Identify the stratified squamous non-keratinized epithelium of oesophagus.
4. Identify the oesophageal (mucous glands) in submucosa.
5. Identify the skeletal and smooth muscles in muscularis externa.
6. Draw a diagram of microanatomy of middle one-third of oesophagus

Function of mucous glands in oesophagus

_____

_____

_____

_____

Three points of identification

_____

_____

_____

_____

_____

_____

Date:

Draw all the layers as in previous diagram with the exception of muscularis externa where both smooth and skeletal muscles have to be drawn.

Date:

SDL NOTES

Date:

CARDIOESOPHAGEAL JUNCTION

Number	Competency	Domain	Level	Core (Y/N)	Teaching/learning method	Assessment method	Number required to certify
AN 52.3	Describe and identify the microanatomical features of cardioesophageal junction, corpus luteum	K/S	SH	Y	Lecture, practical	Written/skill assessment	

- Cardioesophageal junction is the junction of the upper end of stomach (cardiac end) and lower end of oesophagus.
- The stratified squamous epithelium of oesophagus abruptly changes into simple columnar epithelium. There are no goblet cells.
- Gastric pits lined by simple columnar cells are present.
- Lamina propria has tubular glands having columnar cells with few parietal and zymogenic cells at the base of gland.
- Muscularis mucosa has inner circular and outer longitudinal smooth muscle layers.
- Submucosa may have mucous acini apart from loose connective tissue.
- Muscularis externa has inner circular and outer longitudinal smooth muscle layers.
- It is covered by serosa (simple squamous epithelium).

Date:

SPECIFIC LEARNING OBJECTIVES

At the end of the session the student should be able to:

1. Identify cardioesophageal junction under the light microscope.
2. Identify the junction of stratified squamous non-keratinized epithelium and simple columnar epithelium.
3. Identify the four layers: Mucosa, submucosa, muscularis externa and serosa.
4. Identify gastric pits and their cells in lamina propria.
5. Identify mucous glands in submucosa.
6. Draw a diagram of microanatomy of cardioesophageal junction.

Applied importance of cardioesophageal junction

_____

_____

_____

_____

Three points of identification

_____

_____

_____

_____

_____

_____

Date:

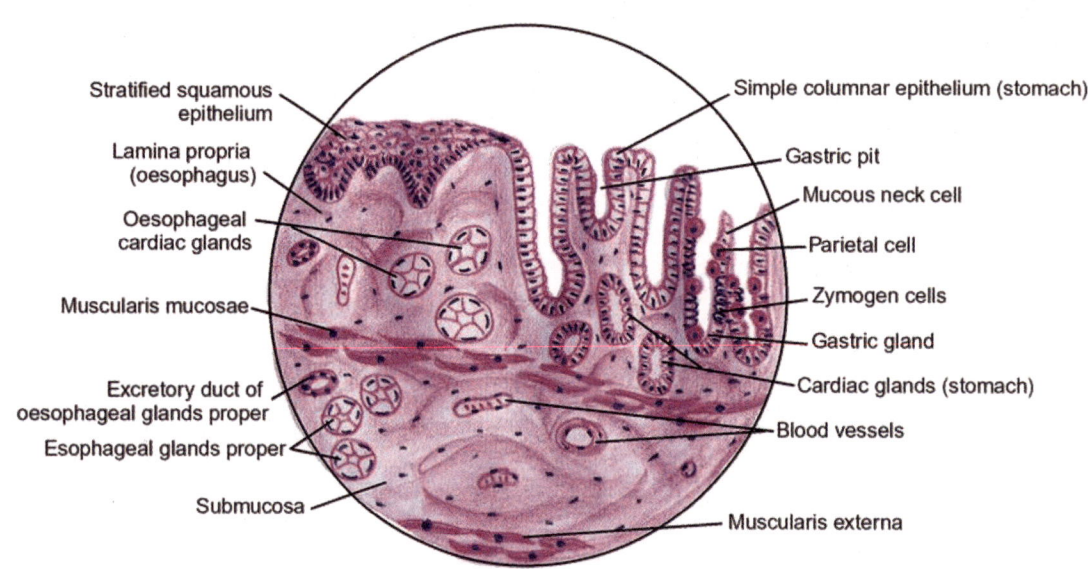

Stratified squamous epithelium

Lamina propria (oesophagus)

Oesophageal cardiac glands

Muscularis mucosae

Excretory duct of oesophageal glands proper

Esophageal glands proper

Submucosa

Simple columnar epithelium (stomach)

Gastric pit

Mucous neck cell

Parietal cell

Zymogen cells

Gastric gland

Cardiac glands (stomach)

Blood vessels

Muscularis externa

STOMACH

TS THROUGH FUNDUS/BODY OF STOMACH

Fundus and Body of Stomach

- Histologically, the fundus and body of stomach are similar.
- Apart from the general layout of GIT, the surface epithelium dips into the lamina propria to form gastric pits. A few (3–7) gastric glands open into each gastric pit (lined by columnar cells).
- Base and body of gastric gland is lined by chief cells/zymogenic/peptic cells. They are pyramidal in shape and have a round nucleus in the centre with granular cytoplasm which stains blue (basophilic). They secrete enzymes.
- Between the chief cells are occasional oxyntic/parietal cells. They secrete H^+ and Cl^- and intrinsic factor. They characteristically appear as large pink cells with large oval nuclei. So they are bright acidophilic cells. These large cells bulge in the lumen of gastric pit and give a beaded appearance.
- Mucous neck cells are present as lining the neck of gastric gland. They are low columnar cells, have mucous and round nuclei.
- Argentaffin cells (triangular cells) at the base of the gastric gland are not stained by H & E staining and require silver salts for staining.
- Muscularis mucosa has thin inner circular and outer longitudinal smooth muscle layers.
- The muscularis externa of body and fundus is different from the general plan of two layers of GIT. It has three layers—innermost oblique, middle circular and outer longitudinal.
- Serosa has squamous cells.

Think and Answer

a. What kind of epithelium will you make in microanatomy of fundus of stomach?

_____

_____

b. What all will you draw in lamina propria of fundus of stomach?

_____

_____

c. How will you draw the muscularis mucosae?

_____

_____

d. What will you draw in submucosa?

_____

_____

e. How many layers of muscles will you draw in muscularis externa of fundus/ body of stomach? How will you draw the different layers?

_____

_____

f. What will be the outermost covering of fundus of stomach?

_____

_____

Date:

FUNDUS/ BODY OF STOMACH (TS)

SPECIFIC LEARNING OBJECTIVES

At the end of the session the student should be able to:

1. Identify the slide under light microscope.
2. Identify the type of epithelium lining the fundus of stomach.
3. Identify the chief cells and oxyntic cells (beaded appearance).
4. Identify the gastric pits and glands.
5. Identify the muscularis mucosa, submucosa, muscularis externa and serosa.
6. Draw a diagram of microanatomy of fundus of stomach.

Function of chief and parietal cells

_____

_____

_____

_____

Three points of identification

_____

_____

_____

_____

_____

_____

Date:

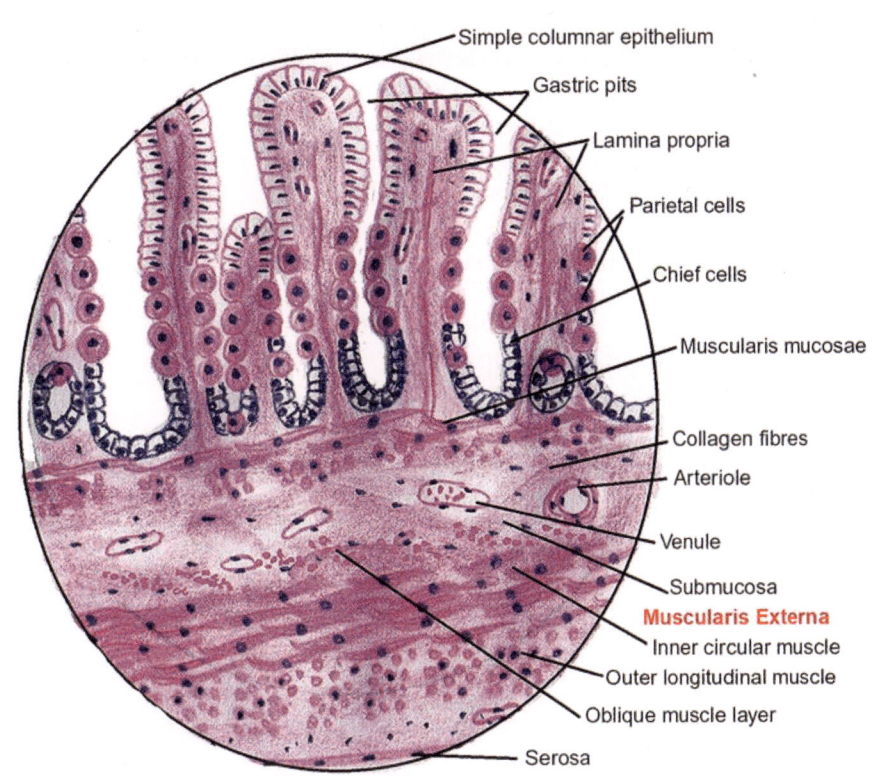

- Simple columnar epithelium
- Gastric pits
- Lamina propria
- Parietal cells
- Chief cells
- Muscularis mucosae
- Collagen fibres
- Arteriole
- Venule
- Submucosa
- **Muscularis Externa**
- Inner circular muscle
- Outer longitudinal muscle
- Oblique muscle layer
- Serosa

Date:

TS THROUGH PYLORUS OF STOMACH

Points of differencesbetween histology of pylorus and fundus/body of stomach

1. Gastric pits are deeper and pyloric glands are shorter with larger lumen.
2. Acini of glands are lightly stained columnar cells, but the nuclei are flattened and situated in the periphery. They secrete mucous and hormone gastrin. They are situated in the lamina propria (same as fundus)
3. Some oxyntic cells may be present.
4. Muscularis externa consists chiefly of thickened circular layer forming the pyloric sphincter.

Now Answer the Following

a. What will be the lining epithelium of pylorus of stomach?

_____

_____

_____

b. What is the characteristic of acini of pyloric glands?

_____

_____

_____

_____

c. What layers of stomach wall will you make?

_____

_____

_____

_____

_____

d. How many layers of muscularis externa will be drawn? Name them.

_____

_____

_____

_____

_____

Date:

SPECIFIC LEARNING OBJECTIVES

At the end of the session the student should be able to:

1. Identify pylorus under the light microscope.
2. Identify all the layers of GIT in the wall of pylorus.
3. Identify pyloric glands
4. Identify thick circular layer of smooth muscles of muscularis externa.
5. Draw a diagram of microanatomy of pylorus.

Function of inner circular layer of muscularis externa in pylorus of stomach

_____

_____

_____

_____

Three points of identification

_____

_____

_____

_____

_____

_____

Date:

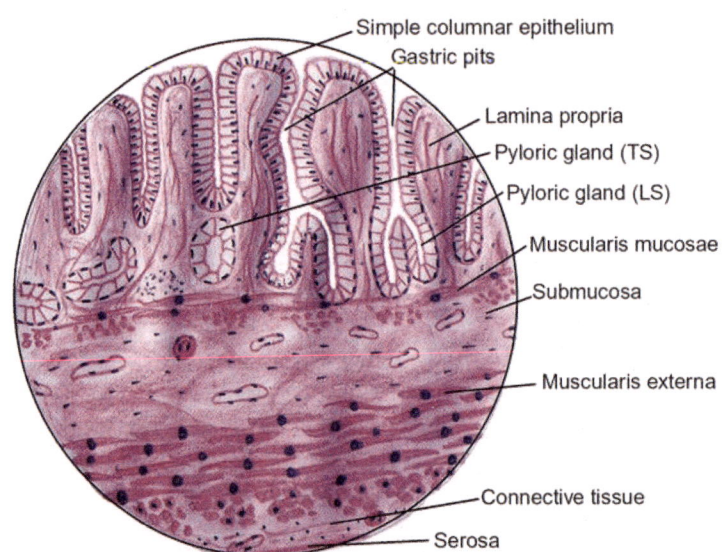

Simple columnar epithelium
Gastric pits
Lamina propria
Pyloric gland (TS)
Pyloric gland (LS)
Muscularis mucosae
Submucosa
Muscularis externa
Connective tissue
Serosa

Date:

SDL NOTES

Date:

SDL NOTES

Date:

INTESTINES

SMALL INTESTINES

- Mucosa—it has permanent folds known as valves of Kerckring. They can be seen with the naked eye. They have mucosa and submucosa.
- Mucosa has intestinal villi which have a core of lamina propria surrounded by columnar epithelium.
- Intestinal glands known as crypts of Lieberkuhn which lie in the lamina propria. They are invaginations of the epithelium (columnar epithelium). They open at the bases of villi. Paneth cells may be seen in the deeper parts of crypts as pink cells because of eosinophilic granules of lysozyme and antibacterial substance. They are pyramidal in shape with basal nuclei
- Lymphocytes may be present as follicles.

DUODENUM

Distinctive Features of Duodenum

- Villi are broad and leaf-shaped with brush border and goblet cells.
- Inner layer of muscularis mucosae sends extensions into the villi. So smooth muscles will be visible in the villi.
- Submucosa has mucous glands known as Brunner's glands or duodenal glands. These have columnar cells with a flat nucleus at the base. Their ducts open into the crypts of Lieberkuhn. They secrete mucous which is alkaline.

Now Answer the Following

Write the kind of epithelium and features of the following in light microscopic picture of duodenum:
1. Lining epithelium is _____
2. Lamina propria has _____
3. Villi are _____ shaped. Their core has _____
4. Muscularis mucosa has _____
5. Submucosa has _____
6. Brunner's glands have _____ cells with _____ nucleus.
7. Muscularis externa has _____ layers consisting of _____
   and _____
8. _____ part of duodenum is not covered by serosa on all sides.
9. Brush border represents _____

Date:

DUODENUM

SPECIFIC LEARNING OBJECTIVES

At the end of the session the student should be able to:

1. Identify duodenum under the light microscope.
2. Identify the four layers of the wall of duodenum.
3. Identify the villi and lining epithelium of duodenum.
4. Identify the submucosa and Brunner's glands present in it.
5. Draw a diagram of microanatomy of duodenum.

Distribution and function of Brunner's glands

_____

_____

_____

_____

Three points of identification

_____

_____

_____

_____

_____

_____

Date:

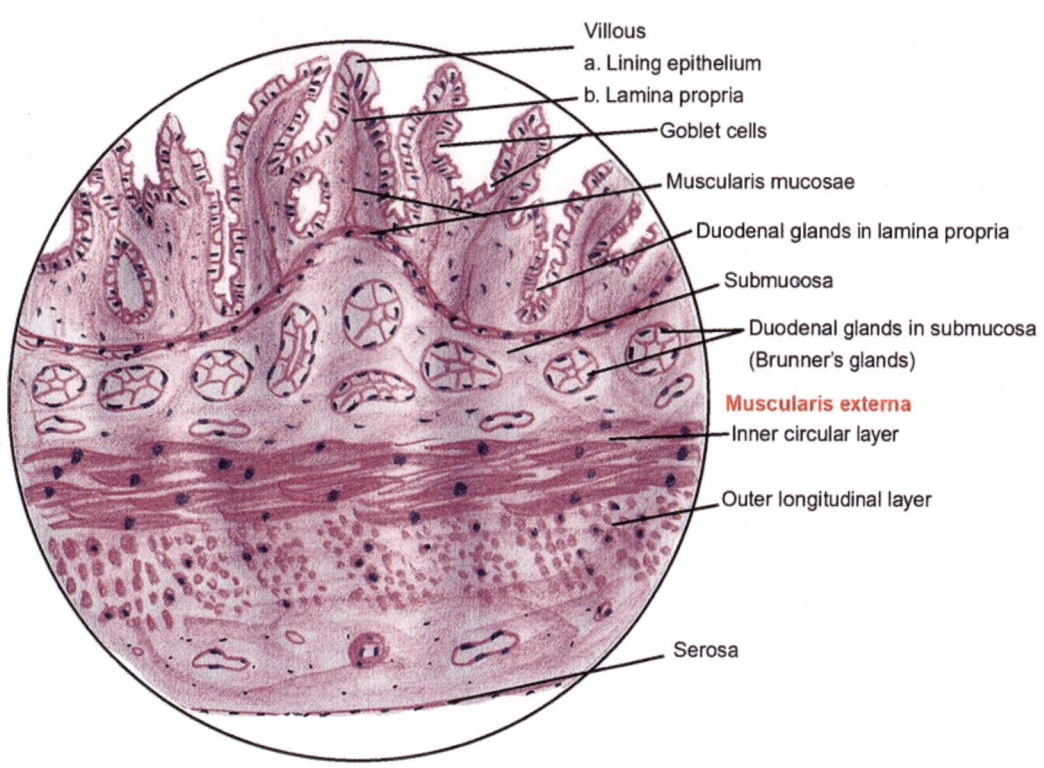

Villous
a. Lining epithelium
b. Lamina propria
Goblet cells
Muscularis mucosae
Duodenal glands in lamina propria
Submuoosa
Duodenal glands in submucosa
(Brunner's glands)
Muscularis externa
Inner circular layer
Outer longitudinal layer
Serosa

Date:

JEJUNUM

SPECIAL FEATURES OF JEJUNUM
- Villi are tongue shaped.
- Special feature is absence of characteristic features of other parts of small intestine, i.e., absence of Brunner's glands and absence of Peyer's patches.
- So if villi are present and other layers of general plan of GIT are seen under the microscope, but the features mentioned above are absent, then it is identified as jejunum.

SPECIFIC LEARNING OBJECTIVES
At the end of the session the student should be able to:
1. Identify jejunum under the light microscope.
2. Identify mucosa, lamina propria, muscularis mucosa, submucosa, muscularis externa and serosa.
3. Identify tongue shaped villi and crypts of Lieberkuhn.
4. Identify the absence of Brunner's glands and Peyer's patches.
5. Draw a diagram of microanatomy of jejunum.

Function of crypts of Lieberkuhn

_____

_____

_____

_____

Three points of identification

_____

_____

_____

_____

_____

_____

Date:

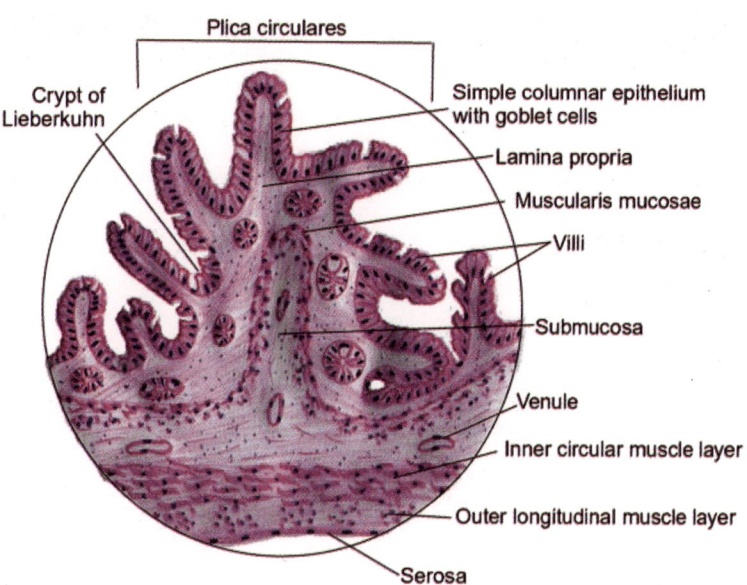

Plica circulares

Crypt of
Lieberkuhn

Simple columnar epithelium
with goblet cells

Lamina propria

Muscularis mucosae

Villi

Submucosa

Venule

Inner circular muscle layer

Outer longitudinal muscle layer

Serosa

Date:

ILEUM

SPECIAL FEATURES OF ILEUM

- Villi are thinner, shorter and finger-shaped.
- Peyer's patches are present in lamina propria. These are lymphoid follicles.

SPECIFIC LEARNING OBJECTIVES

At the end of the session the student should be able to:

1. Identify ileum under the light microscope.
2. Identify the villi and lining epithelium.
3. Identify all the layers of the wall of GIT.
4. Identify Peyer's patches (lymphoid follicles) in lamina propria.
5. Draw a diagram of microanatomy of ileum.

Function of Peyer's patches

_____

_____

_____

_____

Three points of identification

_____

_____

_____

_____

_____

_____

Date:

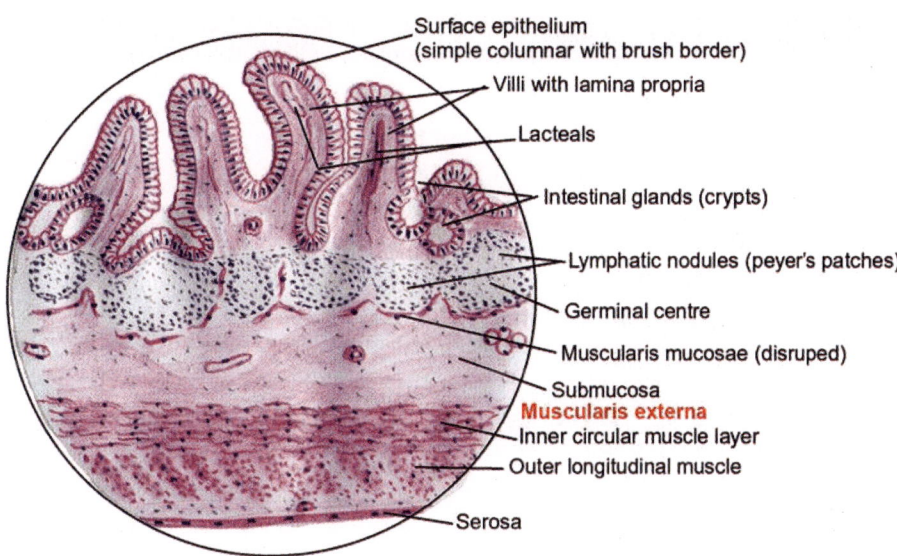

Surface epithelium
(simple columnar with brush border)

Villi with lamina propria

Lacteals

Intestinal glands (crypts)

Lymphatic nodules (peyer's patches)

Germinal centre

Muscularis mucosae (disruped)

Submucosa

Muscularis externa
Inner circular muscle layer

Outer longitudinal muscle

Serosa

Date:

LARGE INTESTINE

MICROSCOPIC FEATURES OF LARGE INTESTINE

- There are no villi or plica circulares as compared from the small intestine.
- The lining epithelium is simple columnar but has numerous goblet cells.
- Microvilli are present which make the outline of columnar cells appear dark pink stained.
- Deep crypts of Lieberkuhn are present. They also have goblet cells.
- Lamina propria has lymphoid follicles.
- Submucosa is the same as the general plan of GIT.
- Muscularis externa has the same two layers but the outer longitudinal layer forms three bands known as taenia coli in addition to forming the outer layer.
- Serosa (mesothelium) + adventitia covering is seen in transverse and sigmoid colon whereas retroperitoneal ascending and descending colon have only adventitia covering.

Answer the Following

1. List the differences between small and large intestines.

Small Intestine	Large Intestine

2. Which muscular coat forms taenia coli?

_____

_____

_____

Date:

VERMIFORM APPENDIX

DIFFERENCES FROM LARGE INTESTINE

- Smaller lumen
- There are no taenia coli
- There are numerous lymphoid follicles in lamina propria which encroach into the submucosa.
- Muscularis mucosa is interrupted and muscularis externa is thin.
- Serosa covers it completely.

Answer the Following

1. How will you differentiate between appendix and fallopian tube under the light microscope?

_____

_____

_____

_____

_____

2. What is the difference between lymphoid follicles of appendix and ileum under microscope?

_____

_____

_____

_____

_____

3. What is the difference between lumen of appendix and vas deferens as seen in microscope?

_____

_____

_____

_____

_____

4. How will you differentiate between the microstructure of appendix and lymph node?

_____

_____

_____

_____

_____

Date:

SPECIFIC LEARNING OBJECTIVES

At the end of the session the student should be able to:

1. Identify vermiform appendix under the light microscope
2. Identify lymphoid follicles in lamina propria and submucosa.
3. Identify the interrupted muscularis mucosae and thin muscularis externa.
4. Identify serosa covering.
5. Differentiate it from microscopic appearance of lymph node.
6. Draw a diagram of microanatomy of vermiform appendix.

Function of appendix

_____

_____

_____

_____

Three points of identification

_____

_____

_____

_____

_____

_____

Date:

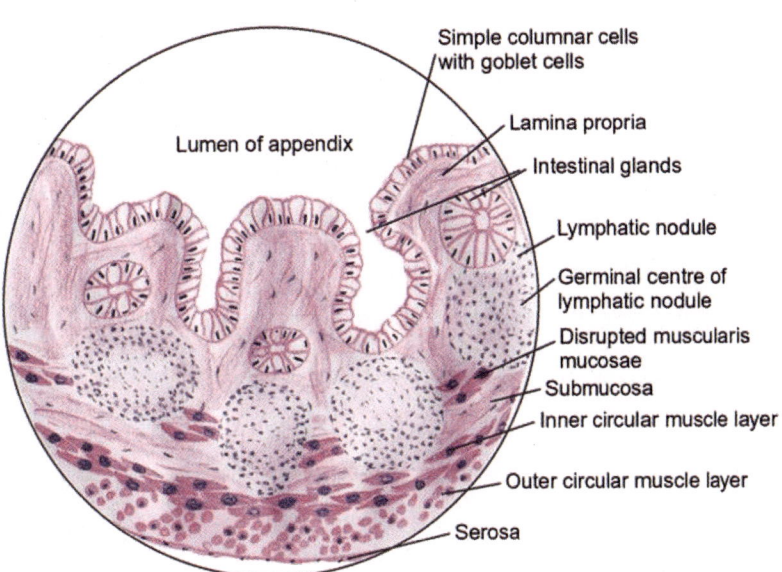

Simple columnar cells with goblet cells

Lumen of appendix

Lamina propria

Intestinal glands

Lymphatic nodule

Germinal centre of lymphatic nodule

Disrupted muscularis mucosae

Submucosa

Inner circular muscle layer

Outer circular muscle layer

Serosa

Date:

COLON

SPECIFIC LEARNING OBJECTIVES

At the end of the session the student should be able to:
1. Identify colon under the light microscope.
2. Identify its lining columnar epithelium along with presence of numerous goblet cells.
3. Identify deep crypts of Lieberkuhn.
4. Appreciate the absence of villi.
5. Thickened longitudinal muscle layer of muscularis externa at three places—taenia coli.
6. Recognize all the layers of wall of GIT.
7. Draw a diagram of microanatomy of colon.

Function of goblet cells

_____

_____

_____

_____

Three points of identification

_____

_____

_____

_____

_____

_____

Date:

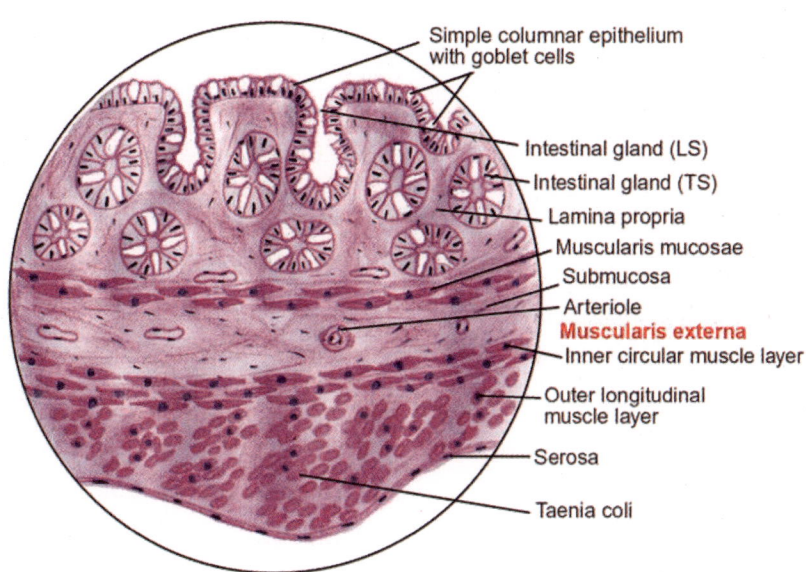

- Simple columnar epithelium with goblet cells
- Intestinal gland (LS)
- Intestinal gland (TS)
- Lamina propria
- Muscularis mucosae
- Submucosa
- Arteriole
- **Muscularis externa**
- Inner circular muscle layer
- Outer longitudinal muscle layer
- Serosa
- Taenia coli

Date:

SDL NOTES

Date:

SDL NOTES

Date:

HEPATOBILIARY SYSTEM

Number	Competency	Domain	Level	Core (Y/N)	Teaching/learning method	Assessment method	Number required to certify
AN 52.1	Describe and identify the microanatomical features of Gastrointestinal system: Oesophagus, fundus of stomach, pylorus of stomach, duodenum, jejunum, ileum, large intestine, appendix, liver gall bladder, pancreas and suprarenal gland	K/S	SH	Y	Lecture, practical	Written/skill assessment	

LIVER

- Liver is covered by Glisson's capsule seen as eosinophilic connective tissue on H & E staining. This extends in the substance of liver and divides it into the characteristic lobules.
- Classical lobule is hexagonal in shape. The hepatocytes in parenchyma are polyhedral in shape. They are arranged in plates seen as radiating from the central vein. They are anastomosing and separated by hepatic sinusoids. Space between hepatocytes and sinusoids is known as space of Disse which lodges hepatic stellate cells called Ito cells (identified by light staining vacuolar appearance due to lipid droplets).
- Sinusoids are lined by phagocytic Kupffer cells (stellate/rounded in shape, difficult to identify under light microscope) and endothelial cells (simple squamous epithelium).
- The angles of hexagon have portal triads consisting of branches of portal artery (lined by endothelium having tunica media with smooth muscles and round lumen), portal vein tributaries (lined by endothelium and having thin tunica media but lumen larger than the artery) and bile ductules (lined by simple cuboidal epithelium). The centre has a central vein.

Date:

SPECIFIC LEARNING OBJECTIVES

At the end of the session the student should be able to:
1. Identify liver under the light microscope.
2. Identify its capsule, hepatocytes and hepatic lobules.
3. Identify the portal triad and its component vessels-hepatic arteriole, hepatic venule, bile ductule.
4. Identify central vein, hepatic sinusoids.
5. Draw a diagram of microanatomy of liver.

Function of sinusoids of liver

_____

_____

_____

_____

Three points of identification

_____

_____

_____

_____

_____

_____

Date:

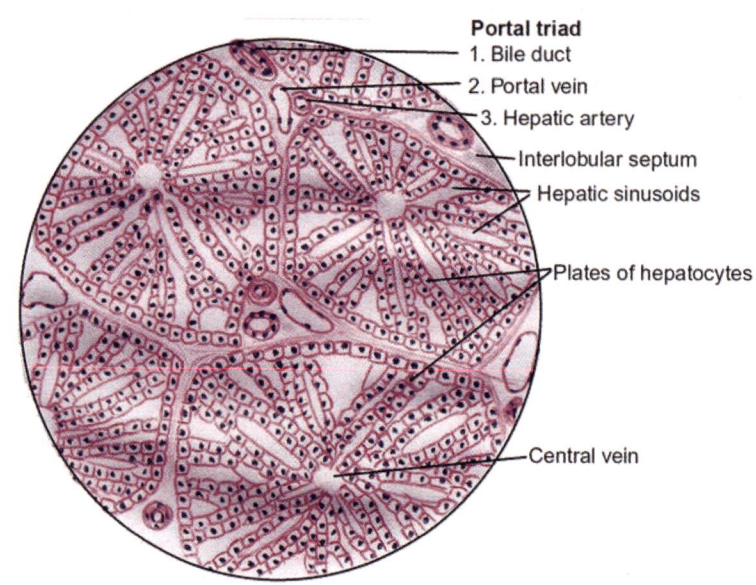

Portal triad
1. Bile duct
2. Portal vein
3. Hepatic artery
Interlobular septum
Hepatic sinusoids
Plates of hepatocytes
Central vein

Date:

PANCREAS

- Pancreas is covered by a thin layer of connective tissue. Numerous septa arise from this and divide the parenchyma into lobules.
- Exocrine part has acini which are serous (like acini of parotid gland).
- Intercalated duct, intralobular duct (simple cuboidal), and interlobular ducts (simple columnar) are seen which finally drain into pancreatic duct.
- Endocrine part has islets of Langerhans which are scattered between exocrine acini. Cells of islets are polyhedral in shape and arranged as cords. Capillaries are seen between the polyhedral cells. Alpha, delta, gamma and PP (Pancreatic polypeptide cells which were formerly known as gamma cells) types of cells of islets of Langerhans cannot be identified in H & E staining. This requires immune-cytochemical methods to be identified.
- The cells of islets stain light and appear pale. Alpha cells have red granules and beta cells have blue granules. They are present in clusters.

Answer the Following

1. Which salivary gland has serous acini?

_____

_____

_____

2. What is the shape of cell and colour of cytoplasm of serous acini?

_____

_____

_____

_____

_____

3. Where is the nucleus located in a cell of serous acinus?

_____

_____

_____

_____

4. How will you differentiate a pancreas from parotid gland on light microscopy?

_____

_____

_____

_____

_____

_____

_____

Date:

SPECIFIC LEARNING OBJECTIVES

At the end of the session the student should be able to:
1. Identify pancreas under the light microscope.
2. Identify lobules and serous acini.
3. Identify islets of Langerhans and capillaries in it.
4. Draw a diagram of microanatomy of pancreas.

Function of serous acinic and islets of Langerhans in pancreas

_____

_____

_____

_____

Three points of identification

_____

_____

_____

_____

_____

_____

Date:

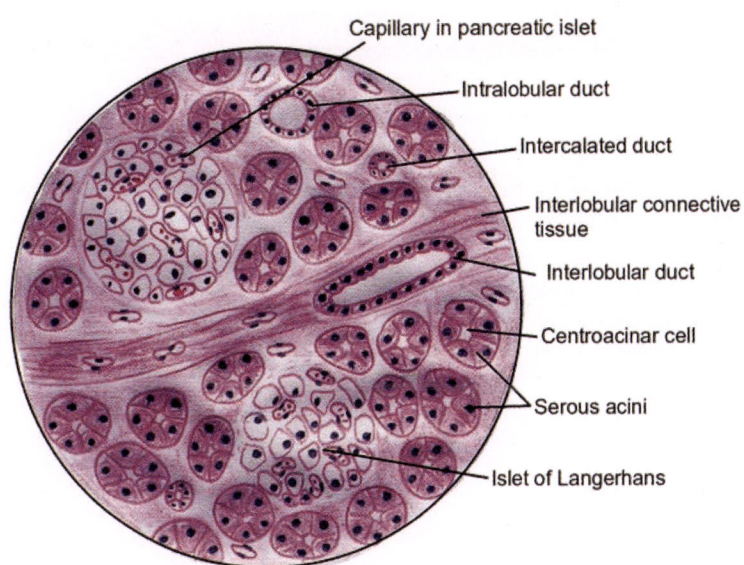

Capillary in pancreatic islet

Intralobular duct

Intercalated duct

Interlobular connective tissue

Interlobular duct

Centroacinar cell

Serous acini

Islet of Langerhans

Date:

GALL BLADDER

- Gall bladder mucosa has temporary folds.
- Its epithelium is of tall columnar cells with nuclei oval in shape and near the base.
- There are no goblet cells in the epithelium.
- Luminal surface of the cells have a dark pink border as seen under the microscope. This is due to microvilli which form brush border.
- Lamina propria is present.
- Muscularis mucosae and glands are absent.
- So outer to the lamina propria there is a fibromuscular layer which represents muscularis externa. So it will have pink staining collagen fibres and spindle shaped smooth muscles with pink cytoplasm and blue central nucleus.
- Outermost layer is of serosa or adventitia.

Think and Answer

1. How will you differentiate the mucosal folds of gall bladder from the villi of small intestine?

_____

_____

_____

_____

2. What is the difference between muscularis externa of general GIT plan and that of gall bladder?

_____

_____

_____

_____

_____

3. What is brush border?

_____

_____

_____

_____

_____

Date:

SPECIFIC LEARNING OBJECTIVES

At the end of the session the student should be able to:
1. Identify gall bladder under the light microscope.
2. Identify the lining epithelium of gall bladder.
3. Identify the absence of muscularis mucosae.
4. Identify the layers of wall of gall bladder.
5. Draw a diagram of microanatomy of gall bladder.

Function of gall bladder

_____

_____

_____

_____

Three points of identification

_____

_____

_____

_____

_____

_____

Date:

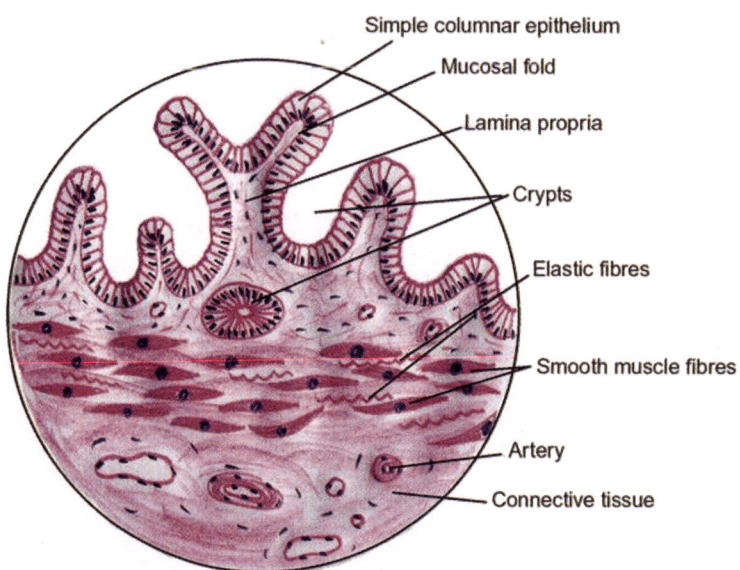

Simple columnar epithelium

Mucosal fold

Lamina propria

Crypts

Elastic fibres

Smooth muscle fibres

Artery

Connective tissue

Date:

SDL NOTES

Date:

SDL NOTES

Date:

URINARY SYSTEM

Number	Competency	Domain	Level	Core (Y/N)	Teaching/learning method	Assessment method	Number required to certify
AN52.2	Describe and identify the microanatomical features of: Urinary system: Kidney, ureter and urinary bladder Male reproductive system: Testis, epididymis, vas deferens, prostate and penis Female reproductive system: Ovary, uterus, uterine tube, cervix, placenta and umbilical cord	K/S	SH	Y	Lecture, practical	Written/skill assessment	

The various structures encountered in the kidney have been mentioned in the schematic diagrams given below. It is advisable to go through each of the given structures and their microscopic characteristic mentioned along with it.

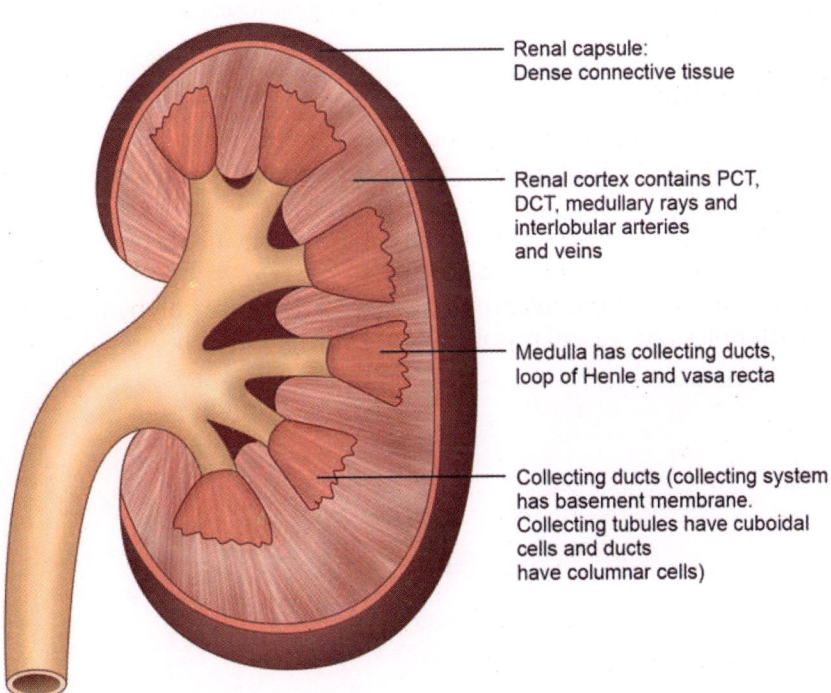

Renal capsule: Dense connective tissue

Renal cortex contains PCT, DCT, medullary rays and interlobular arteries and veins

Medulla has collecting ducts, loop of Henle and vasa recta

Collecting ducts (collecting system has basement membrane. Collecting tubules have cuboidal cells and ducts have columnar cells)

Schematic diagram of LS of Kidney

Date:

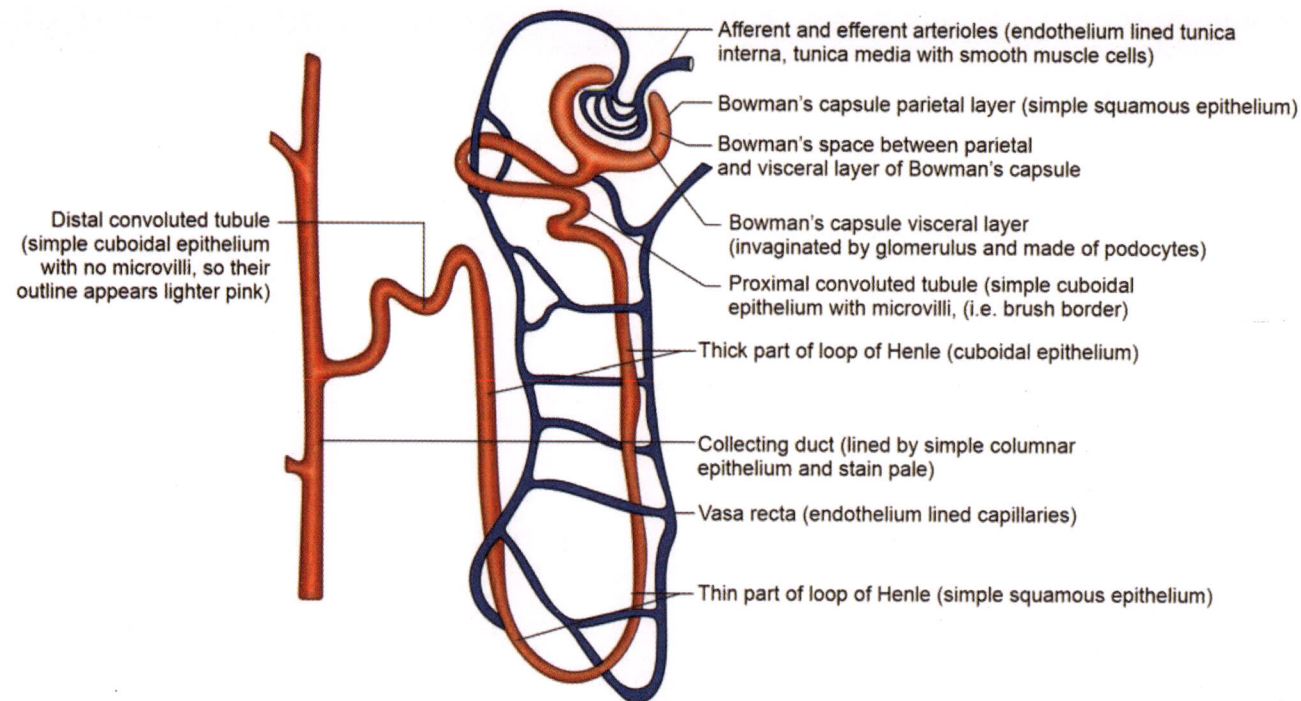

Afferent and efferent arterioles (endothelium lined tunica interna, tunica media with smooth muscle cells)

Bowman's capsule parietal layer (simple squamous epithelium)

Bowman's space between parietal and visceral layer of Bowman's capsule

Bowman's capsule visceral layer (invaginated by glomerulus and made of podocytes)

Proximal convoluted tubule (simple cuboidal epithelium with microvilli, (i.e. brush border)

Thick part of loop of Henle (cuboidal epithelium)

Collecting duct (lined by simple columnar epithelium and stain pale)

Vasa recta (endothelium lined capillaries)

Thin part of loop of Henle (simple squamous epithelium)

Distal convoluted tubule (simple cuboidal epithelium with no microvilli, so their outline appears lighter pink)

Schematic diagram of a nephron and collecting system showing microscopic characteristics on H & E staining

JUXTAGLOMERULAR APPARATUS

It is situated near the glomerulus. It has three components:

1. Macula densa is modified cells in the DCT near the afferent arteriole. The cells are columnar (instead of cuboidal of DCT).

2. Juxtaglomerular cells are modified smooth muscle cells of the tunica media of afferent arterioles of glomerulus. Their cells are large and rounded with spherical nuclei.

3. Lacis cells/cells of polkissen/extraglomerular mesangial cells. They are polyhedral cells between macula densa, afferent and efferent arterioles and vascular pole of kidney.

Date:

KIDNEY

SPECIFIC LEARNING OBJECTIVES

At the end of the session the student should be able to:

1. Identify kidney under the light microscope.
2. Identify cortex having renal corpuscles, PCT (more numerous in number), DCT, and collecting ducts.
3. Indentify medulla having more of collecting ducts, loop of Henle and vasa recta.
4. Identify Bowman's capsule, glomerulus.
5. Appreciate the brush border of PCT.
6. Draw a diagram of microanatomy of kidney.

Distribution and function

_____

_____

_____

_____

Three points of identification

_____

_____

_____

_____

_____

_____

Date:

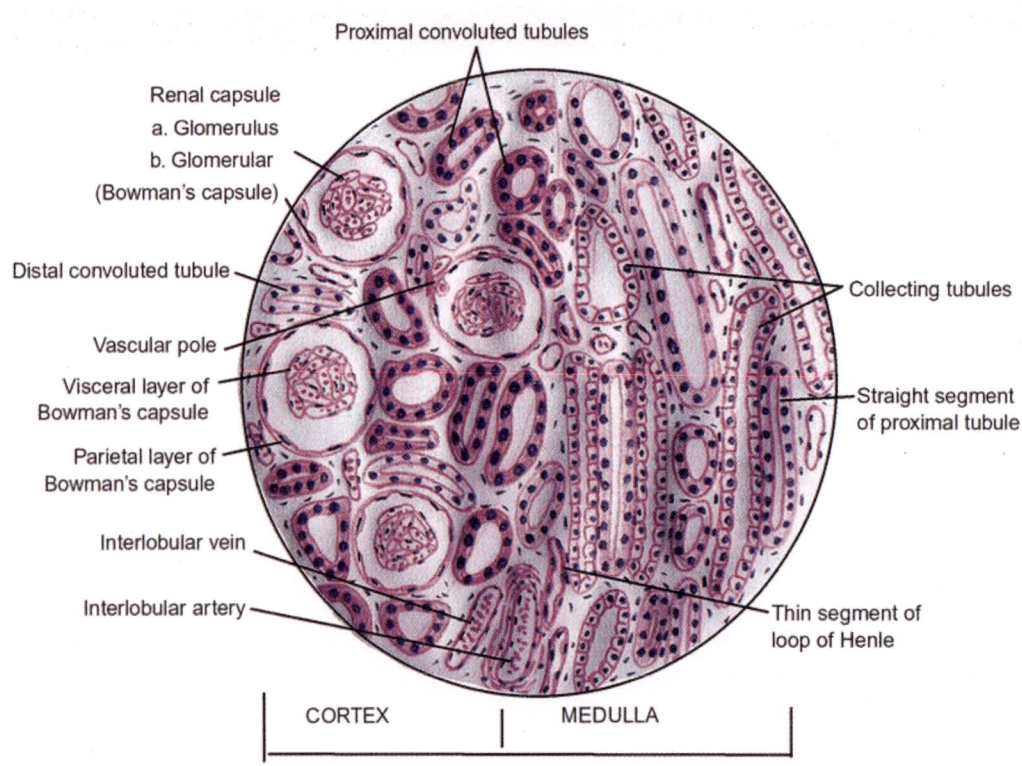

Proximal convoluted tubules

Renal capsule
a. Glomerulus
b. Glomerular
(Bowman's capsule)

Distal convoluted tubule

Vascular pole

Visceral layer of
Bowman's capsule

Parietal layer of
Bowman's capsule

Interlobular vein

Interlobular artery

Collecting tubules

Straight segment
of proximal tubule

Thin segment of
loop of Henle

CORTEX   MEDULLA

Date:

SDL NOTES

Date:

URETER

- The wall of Ureter has three layers—mucosa, muscular layer and adventitia.
- Lumen appears 'star shaped' due to folding of mucosa.
- Epithelium is transitional epithelium.
- Lamina propria lies beneath the epithelium.
- Muscular layer is opposite of general plan of GIT, so it has inner longitudinal and outer circular layer. Lower 1/3rd has a 3rd layer- outermost longitudinal layer.

Think and Answer

1. How many layers of cells are there in the transitional epithelium of ureter?

_____

_____

_____

2. What is the shape of cells of transitional epithelium towards the luminal surface?

_____

_____

_____

3. Is there a basement membrane in transitional epithelium?

_____

_____

_____

_____

4. How will you draw the inner longitudinal layer of muscles in a TS of ureter?

_____

_____

_____

_____

5. How will you draw the outer circular layer of muscles in a TS of ureter?

_____

_____

_____

_____

Date:

SPECIFIC LEARNING OBJECTIVES

At the end of the session the student should be able to:

1. Identify ureter under the light microscope.
2. Appreciate the star-shaped lumen and transitional epithelium.
3. Identify the inner longitudinal and outer circular muscle layer.
4. Draw a diagram of microanatomy of TS of ureter.

Distribution and function

_____

_____

_____

_____

Three points of identification

_____

_____

_____

_____

_____

_____

Date:

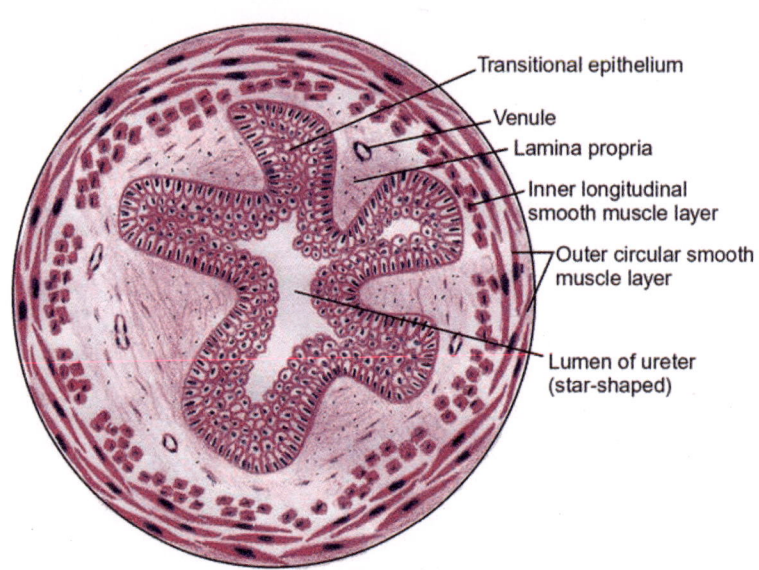

- Transitional epithelium
- Venule
- Lamina propria
- Inner longitudinal smooth muscle layer
- Outer circular smooth muscle layer
- Lumen of ureter (star-shaped)

Date:

URINARY BLADDER

- Mucosa of urinary bladder has folds in relaxed state.
- Mucous membrane has transitional epithelium. (Refer chapter on epithelium). Muscularis mucosae are absent.
- Muscular layer (detrusor muscle) has thick layer of smooth muscles. They are seen to run in different directions. The innermost and outermost layers are oriented more longitudinally whereas the middle layer is more circular. Most of them run obliquely.
- Outermost layer is mostly adventitia except superiorly where there is serosa.

Think and Answer

1. How many layers of cells are there in epithelium of stretched bladder?

_____

_____

_____

2. What happens to the cells when urinary bladder stretches?

_____

_____

_____

_____

3. Which layer of muscles will form the sphincter vesicae?

_____

_____

_____

_____

4. Why is the superior surface of bladder covered with serosa instead of adventitia?

_____

_____

_____

_____

_____

_____

Date:

SPECIFIC LEARNING OBJECTIVES

At the end of the session the student should be able to:
1. Indentify urinary bladder under the light microscope.
2. Identify transitional epithelium.
3. Identify muscular layers.
4. Identify serosa/adventitia.
5. Draw the diagram of microanatomy of urinary bladder.

Function of transitional epithelium

_____

_____

_____

_____

Three points of identification

_____

_____

_____

_____

_____

_____

Date:

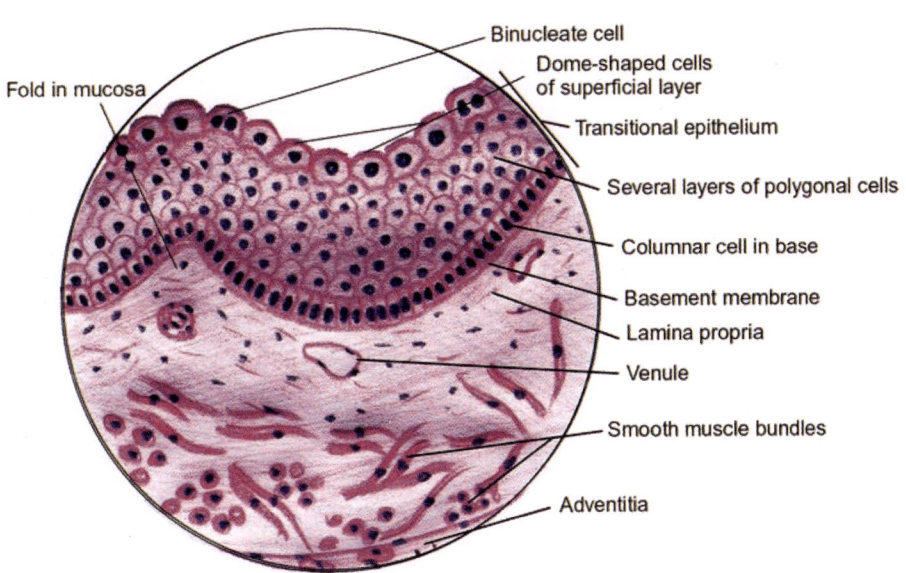

- Binucleate cell
- Dome-shaped cells of superficial layer
- Fold in mucosa
- Transitional epithelium
- Several layers of polygonal cells
- Columnar cell in base
- Basement membrane
- Lamina propria
- Venule
- Smooth muscle bundles
- Adventitia

Date:

SDL NOTES

Date:

SDL NOTES

Date:

REPRODUCTIVE SYSTEM

Number	Competency	Domain	Level	Core (Y/N)	Teaching/learning method	Assessment method	Number required to certify
AN52.2	Describe and identify the microanatomical features of: Urinary system: Kidney, ureter and urinary bladder Male reproductive system: Testis, epididymis, vas deferens, prostate and penis Female reproductive system: Ovary, uterus, uterine tube, cervix, placenta and umbilical cord	K/S	SH	Y	Lecture, practical	Written/skill assessment	

MALE REPRODUCTIVE SYSTEM

Testis

- The three coverings of testis from outside inwards are tunica vaginalis, tunica albuginea and tunica vasculosa. Tunica vaginalis is a lining of serosa all around the testis except at the posterior border.
- Tunica albuginea is a layer of dense connective tissue. It forms the mediastinum testis at its posterior part. Its septa extend anteriorly dividing the testis into lobules.
- Each lobule is lined by a vascular layer called the tunica vasculosa.
- Inside each lobule are seminiferous tubules, interstitial cells of Leydig and loose connective tissue.
- Near the posterior part the seminiferous tubules join to form a network of tubules called rete testis.
- Seminiferous tubules:
  o They are lined by a special stratified seminiferous epithelium. The cells found in it are spermatogenic cells (form sperms) which are seen to be in various stages of spermatogenesis; and Sertoli cells (supporting cells).
  o The stages of cells of spermatogenesis that can be seen are:
    1. Spermatogonia in contact with the basement membrane. They stain lightly.
    2. Primary spermatocytes—largest germ cells
    3. Secondary spermatocytes—smaller than primary spermatocytes. They are rarely seen in histology slides because of their short lifespan.
    4. Spermatids lie towards the lumen.
    5. Spermatozoa lie in the lumen and are flagellated.
  o Sertoli cells are pyramidal in shape with oval nucleus. They are tall cells and extend from the basement membrane to the lumen of seminiferous tubule. Their cytoplasm is eosinophilic (stains pink) and granular.
- Leydig cells are present in clusters between adjacent seminiferous tubules. They are polygonal cells with round nuclei.

Date:

TESTIS

SPECIFIC LEARNING OBJECTIVES

At the end of the session the student should be able to:
1. Identify testis under light microscope.
2. Identify seminiferous tubules.
3. Identify spermatogonia, Sertoli cells, spermatocytes, and spermatids.
4. Identify Leydig cells.
5. Draw a diagram of microanatomy of testis.

Functions of Sertoli and Leydig cells

_____

_____

_____

_____

Three points of identification

_____

_____

_____

_____

_____

_____

_____

Date:

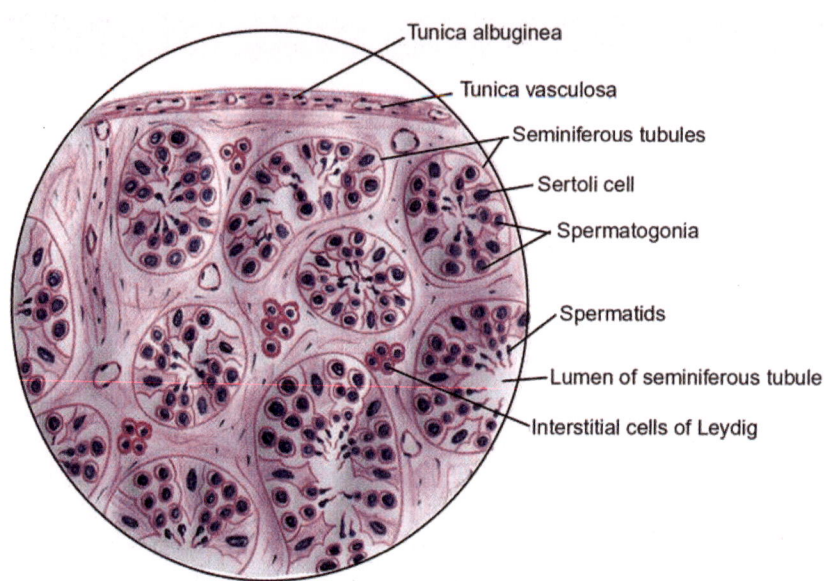

- Tunica albuginea
- Tunica vasculosa
- Seminiferous tubules
- Sertoli cell
- Spermatogonia
- Spermatids
- Lumen of seminiferous tubule
- Interstitial cells of Leydig

Date:

EPIDIDYMIS

- A TS through epididymis shows numerous tubules of different sizes.
- The lining of these tubules is of pseudostratified columnar epithelium.
- They rest on a basement membrane and have smooth muscle fibres arranged around the tubules.
- Luminal surface of the columnar cells have non motile stereocilia.
- Lumen shows spermatozoa within it. (Function of epididymis is storage of sperms and helping in their maturation.)
- Columnar cells absorb testicular fluid and remove degenerating sperms.

Revise Previous Chapters and Answer the Following

1. What is the characteristic feature of pseudostratified columnar epithelium?

_____

_____

_____

_____

2. How will you differentiate between pseudostratified columnar epithelium of respiratory system from that of epididymis?

_____

_____

_____

_____

_____

3. What is the role of smooth muscle fibres around the tubules?

_____

_____

_____

_____

4. What is the difference between stereocilia and cilia?

_____

_____

_____

_____

_____

Date:

SPECIFIC LEARNING OBJECTIVES

At the end of the session the student should be able to:

1. Identify epididymis under the light microscope.
2. Identify pseudostratified columnar epithelium of epididymis.
3. Identify stereocilia.
4. Identify spermatids in the lumen.
5. Draw a diagram of microanatomy of epididymis.

Function of stereocilia in epididymis

_____

_____

_____

_____

Three points of identification

_____

_____

_____

_____

_____

_____

Date:

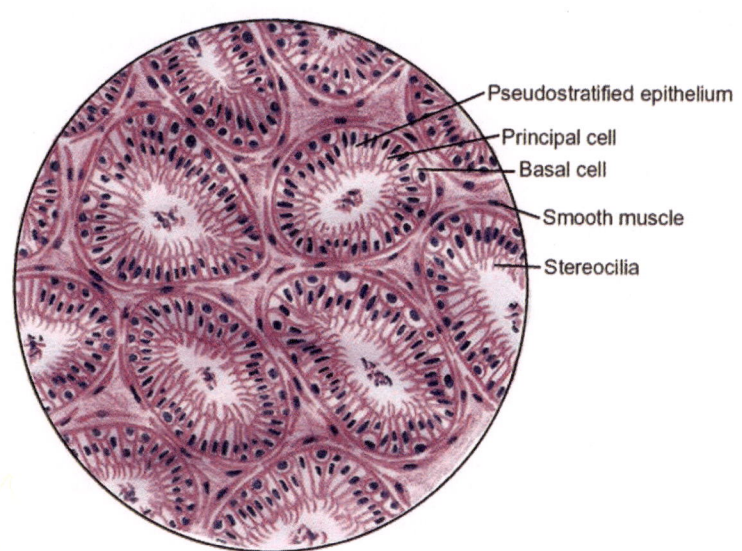

- Pseudostratified epithelium
- Principal cell
- Basal cell
- Smooth muscle
- Stereocilia

Date:

VAS DEFERENS/DUCTUS DEFERENS

- It has a star-shaped lumen as seen under the light microscope.
- It has three layers: inner mucous membrane, middle muscular coat, outer fibrous coat.
- Epithelium is pseudostratified columnar epithelium in the distal part and simple ciliated columnar in the proximal part.
- Lamina propria has elastic fibres which cause the epithelium to be thrown into folds. So the lumen appears star-shaped.
- Middle muscular coat is thick and has three layers: inner and outer are longitudinal muscle fibres and middle layer has circular muscle fibres. The inner longitudinal layer is present in the proximal part of vas deferens.
- Outermost is the adventitia with blood vessels and nerves.
- The whole vas deferens can be seen in one field in low power.

Think and Answer

1. What is the appearance of the shape of lumen of ureter under the light microscope?

_____

_____

_____

2. How will you differentiate between a slide of ureter and vas deferens under the light microscope?

_____

_____

_____

_____

4. What are the examples of tissues with pseudostratified columnar epithelium?

_____

_____

_____

_____

_____

_____

Date:

VAS DEFERENS

SPECIFIC LEARNING OBJECTIVES

At the end of the session the student should be able to:

1. Identify vas deferens under the light microscope.
2. Identify the lining epithelium and star-shaped lumen.
3. Identify layers of muscular coat.
4. Draw a diagram of microanatomy of vas deferens.

Function of vas deferens

Three points of identification

Date:

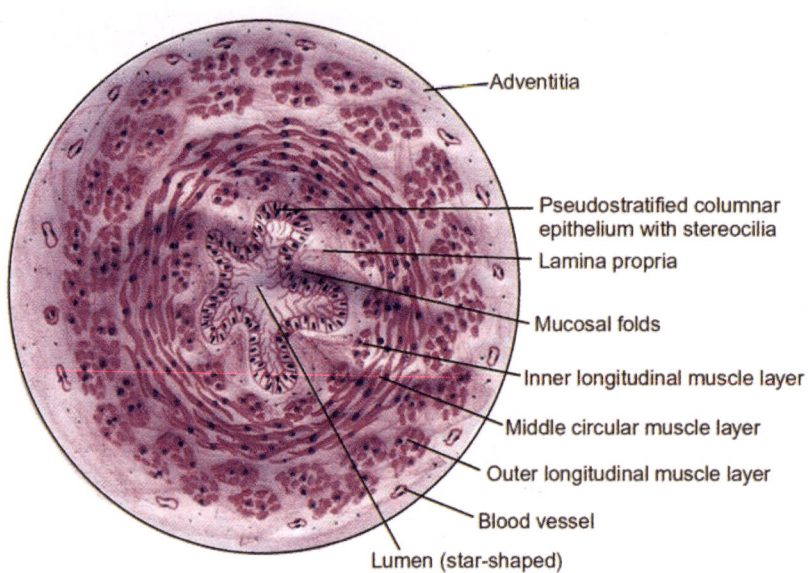

Adventitia

Pseudostratified columnar epithelium with stereocilia

Lamina propria

Mucosal folds

Inner longitudinal muscle layer

Middle circular muscle layer

Outer longitudinal muscle layer

Blood vessel

Lumen (star-shaped)

Date:

PROSTATE

- Prostate is traversed by prostatic urethra. So this part of urethra has three layers: mucosa, submucosa and muscle layer. Mucosa has pseudostratified columnar epithelium. It has recesses in which mucosal glands open. Submucosa has loose connective tissue and submucosal glands which have short ducts which open in the urethra. The muscle coat consists of inner longitudinal and outer circular layer of smooth muscles. All this is in the central zone of prostate.
- An adult prostate consists of tubuloalveolar glands in a fibromuscular tissue. These are main prostatic glands found in the peripheral zone. They have long ducts lined by bilaminar epithelium having columnar cell layer and cuboidal cell layer. These ducts open into the prostatic urethra.
- The glandular part is not well-developed before puberty and degenerates in old age.
- Glandular tissue appears as follicles lined by columnar epithelium. The epithelium is pseudostratified in active glands. This epithelium is characteristically thrown into numerous folds. Near the base there are basal cells responsible for regeneration of epithelium.
- Amyloid bodies/corpora amylacea are seen within the alveoli of follicles in older age. They appear as eosinophilic, lamellated round masses. They are made of glycoprotein.
- The fibromuscular tissue has collagen fibres and smooth muscle. They form septa between glandular follicles.
- Prostate is surrounded by fibrous capsule having numerous veins and parasympathetic ganglion cells.

Date:

SPECIFIC LEARNING OBJECTIVES

At the end of the session the student should be able to:

1. Identify prostate under the light microscope.
2. Identify glandular follicles lined by columnar epithelium.
3. Appreciate the numerous mucosal folds of glandular follicles.
4. Identify collagen fibres and smooth muscle fibres between follicles.
5. Identify corpora amylacea in the follicles.
6. Identify prostatic urethra, if present in section.
7. Draw a diagram of microanatomy of prostate.

Function of glandular follicles of prostate

_____

_____

_____

_____

Three points of identification

_____

_____

_____

_____

_____

_____

Date:

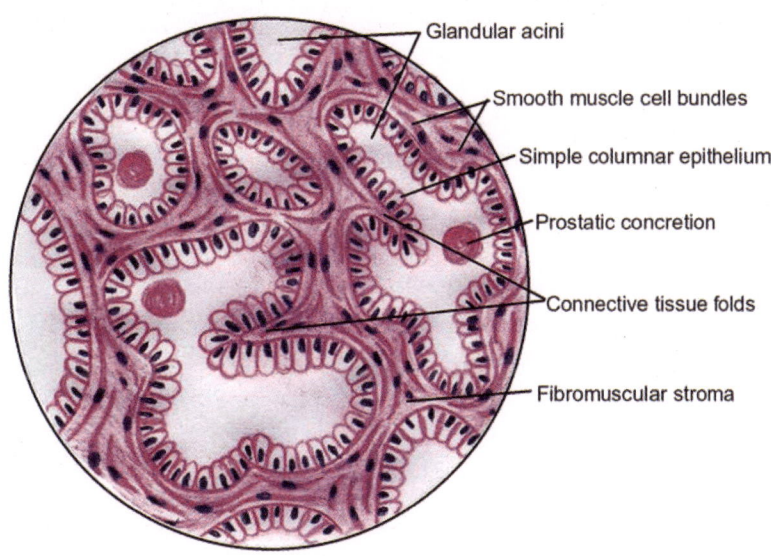

Glandular acini

Smooth muscle cell bundles

Simple columnar epithelium

Prostatic concretion

Connective tissue folds

Fibromuscular stroma

Date:

PENIS

- The outermost covering of penis is thin skin. Hair follicles are present at the root of penis, the rest of the penis being devoid of hair follicles.
- The dermis has smooth muscles and dilated venous spaces.
- There are three cavernous tissues—two corpora cavernosa on the dorsal side and one corpus spongiosum on the ventral side.
- Corpus cavernosum is surrounded by fibrous (collagen and elastic) covering known as tunica albuginea. There are spaces (caverns) which are enclosed by connective tissues and smooth muscle fibres forming trabeculae. Caverns are vascular spaces lined by endothelial cells. There are arterioles and venules.
- Corpus spongiosum has finer trabeculae and narrower arterioles. Throughout the length of corpus spongiosum is the spongy urethra which traverses the penis. Spongy urethra is lined by pseudostratified columnar epithelium except near the terminal part where it is lined by stratified squamous epithelium. The fibrous sheath surrounding the corpus spongiosum is thinner.
- A common fibrous sheath surrounds the corpora cavernosa and corpus spongiosum.

Date:

SPECIFIC LEARNING OBJECTIVES

At the end of the session the student should be able to:

1. Identify penis under the light microscope.
2. Identify corpora cavernosa and corpus spongiosum.
3. Identify the urethra in corpus spongiosum.
4. Identify tunica albuginea.
5. Identify the epidermis and dermis layers of skin of penis.
6. Identify the smooth muscle fibres in dermis.
7. Draw the diagram of microanatomy of penis.

Function of corpora cavernosa and corpus spongiosum

_____

_____

_____

_____

Three points of identification

_____

_____

_____

_____

_____

_____

Date:

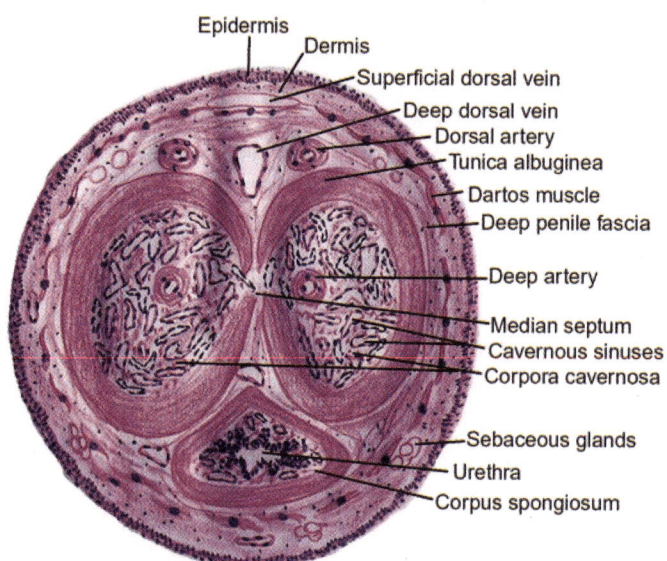

Epidermis
Dermis
Superficial dorsal vein
Deep dorsal vein
Dorsal artery
Tunica albuginea
Dartos muscle
Deep penile fascia
Deep artery
Median septum
Cavernous sinuses
Corpora cavernosa
Sebaceous glands
Urethra
Corpus spongiosum

Date:

SDL NOTES

Date:

SDL NOTES

Date:

FEMALE REPRODUCTIVE SYSTEM

OVARY

- Ovary is the organ responsible for production of ova and hormones of female reproductive system.
- The germinal epithelium producing primordial follicles and ultimately ova is derived from its epithelial covering. This means that the serosal covering of ovary is modified to cuboidal epithelium to form the germinal epithelium.
- The outer cortex of ovary has follicles in different stages of development, viz. primordial follicle, primary follicle, secondary follicle, Graafian follicle, corpus luteum and atretic follicles.
- Apart from the follicles cortex has highly cellular connective tissue stroma.
- The inner medulla has loose connective tissue containing blood vessels, elastic fibres and few smooth muscle fibres.

Histological appearance of the various stages is as follows:

- **Primordial follicle:**
  o Primary oocyte surrounded by simple squamous epithelium.
- **Primary follicle:**
  o Larger oocyte surrounded by cuboidal epithelium. Between the two is the zona pellucida.
  o On further development the cuboidal follicular cell layer becomes multilayered. These follicular cells are called granulosa cells. They are surrounded by a thick basal lamina which appears eosinophilic on H & E staining.
  o Outside this lamina there are stromal cells of the ovary which differentiate into cuboidal cells layer—theca interna and outer fibrous layer—theca externa.
- **Secondary follicle:**
  o Initially numerous fluid filled cavities appear between the follicular cells. These fuse together to form a single cavity called antrum. The liquid within it (liquor folliculi) is not stained by H & E staining, so it appears empty.
  o Granulosa cells at the side of antrum away from oocyte are known as membrana granulosa.
  o Granulosa cells at the side of antrum adjacent to oocyte are known as cumulus oophoricus/cumulus ovaricus.
- **Graafian follicle:**
  o The features of mature Graafian follicle as seen under the microscope are the same as secondary follicle with single antrum with the following differences:
  o Antrum is much larger.
  o The feature not visible under the light microscope is the completion of 1st meiotic division and formation of secondary oocyte. So the oocyte is now known as secondary oocyte.

Date:

OVARY

SPECIFIC LEARNING OBJECTIVES

At the end of the session the student should be able to:

1. Identify ovary under the light microscope.
2. Identify germinal epithelium.
3. Identify cortex and medulla.
4. Identify primordial, primary and secondary follicles.
5. Identify Graafian follicle and its components.
6. Identify corpus luteum, if present.
7. Draw a diagram of microanatomy of ovary.

Function of Graafian follicle

_____

_____

_____

_____

Three points of identification

_____

_____

_____

_____

_____

_____

Date:

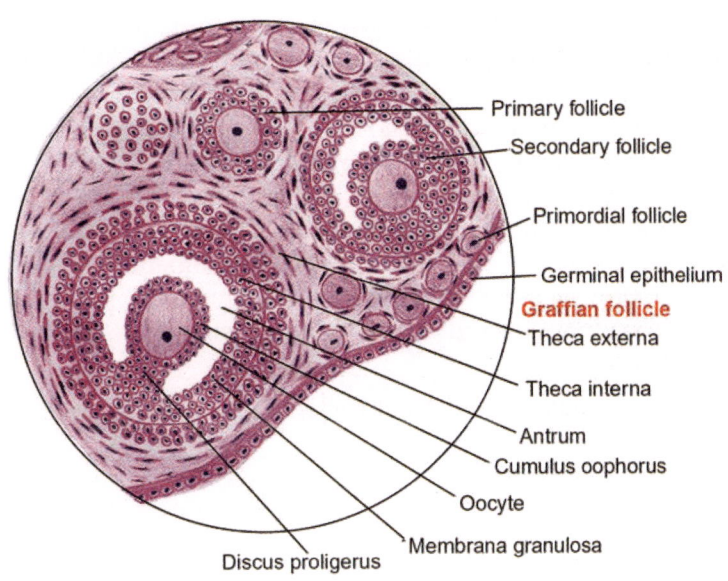

- Primary follicle
- Secondary follicle
- Primordial follicle
- Germinal epithelium
- **Graffian follicle**
- Theca externa
- Theca interna
- Antrum
- Cumulus oophorus
- Oocyte
- Membrana granulosa
- Discus proligerus

Date:

UTERUS

- The wall of uterus has three layers from within outwards: endometrium, myometrium and serosa or adventitia.
- Endometrium has simple columnar epithelium with lamina propria underneath it.
- Lamina propria has simple tubular glands called endometrial glands.
- The deeper basal parts of these glands are not shed in menstruation. This part is called stratum basale. The superficial part of endometrium is called stratum functionale which is shed during menstruation.
- Myometrium is the thickest layer of uterine wall. The bundles of smooth muscle fibres run in different directions. There are blood vessels present between the bundles of smooth muscle.
- Adventitia (on the part of uterus not covered by peritoneum) or serosa (on the part of uterus covered by peritoneum) is the outermost layer.

Proliferative phase (from 4th to 14th day of menstrual cycle)
- Stratum functionale regenerates from stratum basale.
- Thickness of stratum functionale increases.
- Length of endometrial glands increases and spiral artery also increases in length.

Secretory phase (14th to 28th day of menstrual cycle)
- Thickness of endometrium becomes double of proliferative phase.
- Glands become coiled giving the 'saw tooth appearance' in sections. The spiral arteries become coiled and increase in length and span the whole length of stratum functionale.

Menstrual phase (1st to 4th day of menstrual cycle)
- The whole stratum functionale is shed.
- Stratum basale and its arteries remain.

Date:

UTERUS (PROLIFERATIVE PHASE)

SPECIFIC LEARNING OBJECTIVES

At the end of the session the student should be able to:

1. Identify uterus (proliferative phase) under the light microscope.
2. Identify epithelium and its columnar epithelium.
3. Identify lamina propria and tubular endometrial glands.
4. Identify myometrium and blood vessels in it.
5. Draw a diagram of microanatomy of proliferative phase of uterus.

Function of deciduas basalis

_____

_____

_____

_____

Three points of identification

_____

_____

_____

_____

_____

_____

Date:

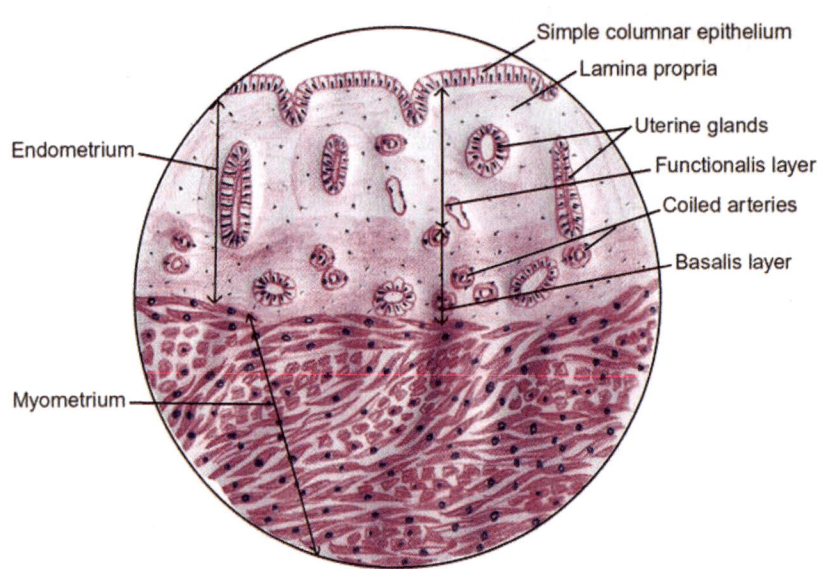

Simple columnar epithelium

Lamina propria

Endometrium

Uterine glands

Functionalis layer

Coiled arteries

Basalis layer

Myometrium

Date:

UTERUS (SECRETORY PHASE)

SPECIFIC LEARNING OBJECTIVES

At the end of the session the student should be able to:

1. Identify uterus (secretory phase) under the light microscope.
2. Identify endometrium, myometrium, adventitia/serosa.
3. Identify coiled tubular endometrial glands by their 'saw-tooth appearance'.
4. Appreciate the greater thickness of endometrium.
5. Identify arteries between muscle bundles and lamina propria.
6. Draw a diagram of microanatomy of secretory phase of uterus.

Function of endometrial glands

_____

_____

_____

_____

Three points of identification

_____

_____

_____

_____

_____

_____

Date:

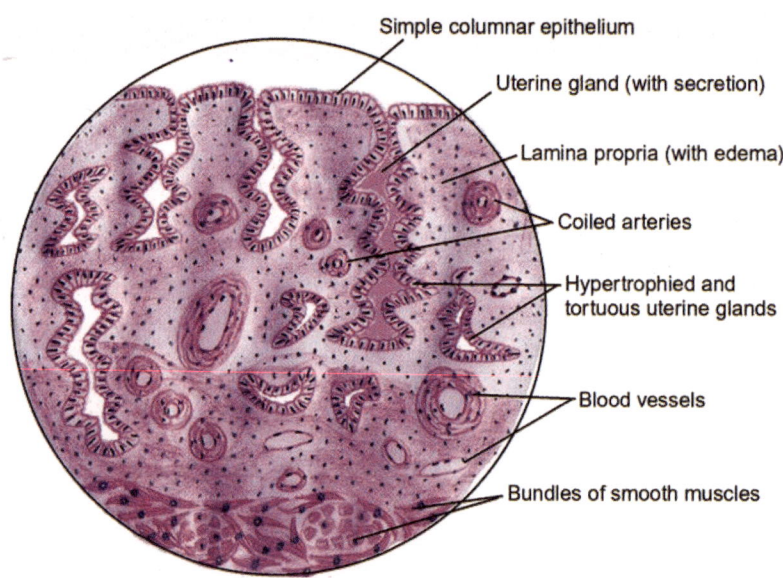

Simple columnar epithelium

Uterine gland (with secretion)

Lamina propria (with edema)

Coiled arteries

Hypertrophied and tortuous uterine glands

Blood vessels

Bundles of smooth muscles

Date:

CERVIX

- A section of cervix shows mucosal epithelium, lamina propria and connective tissue.
- Mucosal epithelium of cervical canal is simple columnar.
- There are cervical glands in lamina propria which open on the epithelium.
- Beyond the external os the simple columnar epithelium changes to non-keratinized squamous epithelium and continues over the outer surface of vaginal part of cervix.
- A few smooth muscle fibres may be seen, but there is no muscular layer.

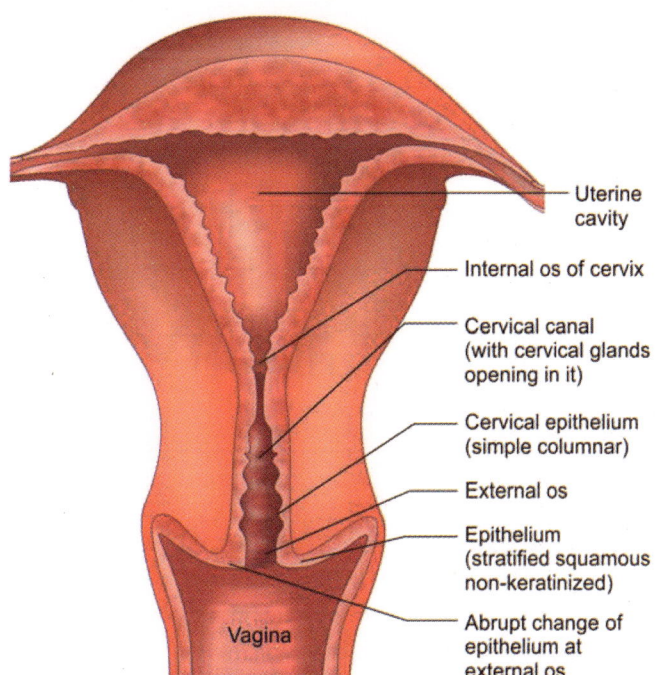

- Uterine cavity
- Internal os of cervix
- Cervical canal (with cervical glands opening in it)
- Cervical epithelium (simple columnar)
- External os
- Epithelium (stratified squamous non-keratinized)
- Abrupt change of epithelium at external os

Vagina

Date:

SPECIFIC LEARNING OBJECTIVES

At the end of the session the student should be able to:

1. Identify cervix under the light microscope.
2. Identify cervical glands.
3. Identify simple columnar epithelium of cervical canal and stratified squamous non-keratinized epithelium of outer surface of cervix and the abrupt change of epithelium at external os.
4. Draw a diagram of microanatomy of cervix.

Function of cervical glands

_____

_____

_____

_____

Three points of identification

_____

_____

_____

_____

_____

_____

Date:

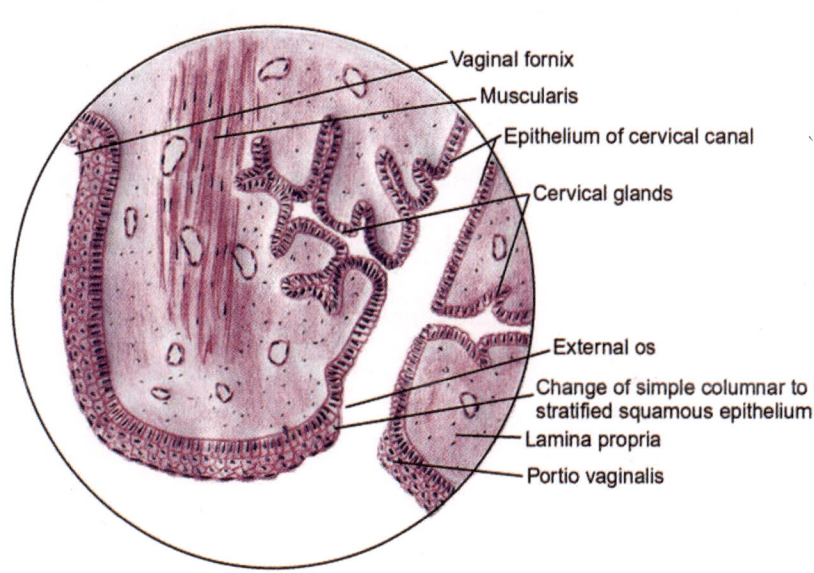

Vaginal fornix

Muscularis

Epithelium of cervical canal

Cervical glands

External os

Change of simple columnar to
stratified squamous epithelium

Lamina propria

Portio vaginalis

Date:

FALLOPIAN TUBE/UTERINE TUBE

- Histologically there are three layers in the wall of fallopian tube—mucosa, muscular layer and serosa.
- The characteristic appearance of mucosa is its numerous folds projecting into the lumen. They appear to obscure the lumen.
- Lining epithelium has ciliated simple columnar cells resting on basement membrane. Non-ciliated cells called peg cells are also present.
- Lamina propria lies beneath the epithelium. It has loose connective tissue with fibroblast cells.
- There is no muscularis mucosa.
- Muscular layer has inner circular and outer longitudinal smooth muscle layers.
- Serosa is the outermost layer made up of mesothelium.

Answer the Following

1. What is the function of cilia in fallopian tube?

_____

_____

_____

2. What is the function of clear or peg cells?

_____

_____

_____

_____

3. What is the role of muscular layer in fallopian tube?

_____

_____

_____

_____

_____

Date:

SPECIFIC LEARNING OBJECTIVES

At the end of the session the student should be able to:
1. Identify fallopian tube under the light microscope.
2. Identify mucosal folds projecting in the lumen.
3. Identify simple columnar ciliated epithelium along with non-ciliated cells in the epithelium.
4. Identify lamina propria.
5. Identify muscular layer—inner circular and outer longitudinal.
6. Draw a diagram of microanatomy of fallopian tube/uterine tube/oviduct.

Function of cilia in uterine tube

_____

_____

_____

_____

Three points of identification

_____

_____

_____

_____

_____

_____

Date:

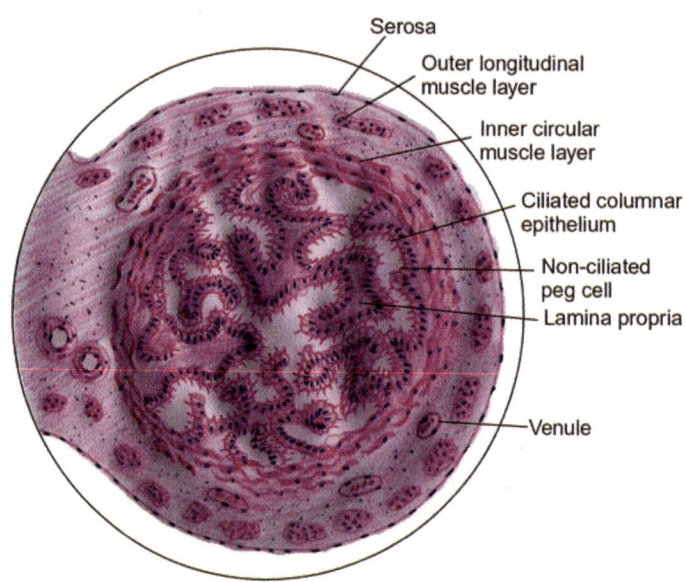

Serosa

Outer longitudinal
muscle layer

Inner circular
muscle layer

Ciliated columnar
epithelium

Non-ciliated
peg cell

Lamina propria

Venule

Date:

PLACENTA

Placenta is the organ which connects the foetus to the mother. It is disc-shaped with a convex maternal and a concave smooth foetal surface. Foetal surface is lined by chorionic plate and maternal surface exhibits cotyledons due to placental septa.

It is better to study development of placenta before studying the microscopic structure. Presuming that it has been studied we proceed with the details of microscopic anatomy.

There are three stages in the development of villi. They are as follows:

1. **Primary villus:** Central core is of cytotrophoblast which is surrounded by syncytiotrophoblast.
2. **Secondary villus:** Mesoderm is at the core, which is then surrounded by cytotrophoblast and then syncytiotrophoblast.
3. **Tertiary villus:** Blood vessels enter the central core of mesoderm. So there is loose connective tissue with foetal capillaries, and phagocytic cells called **Hofbauer cells.** This is then surrounded by cytotrophoblast, and syncytiotrophoblast.

- In a section of placenta we can see the decidua basalis towards the maternal side. It has uterine glands, blood vessels and some smooth muscle fibres.
- The foetal side has amnion and chorionic plate.
- In between are the chorionic villi—anchoring stem villi, primary villi, secondary villi and tertiary villi.
- Cytotrophoblast cells take up light basophilic stain and syncytiotrophoblast stains strongly basophilic on H & E staining.
- **Placental barrier** can be seen comprising of:
  o Syncytiotrophoblast cells
  o Basement membrane of cytotrophoblast cells
  o Basement membrane of foetal capillaries
  o Endothelial cells.

Date:

SPECIFIC LEARNING OBJECTIVES

At the end of the session the student should be able to:

1. Identify placenta under the light microscope.
2. Identify stem, primary, secondary, tertiary villi, as the case may be.
3. Identify cytotrophoblast, syncytiotrophoblast and mesodermal core.
4. Identify foetal capillaries in villi and maternal RBCs in between villi.
5. Identify the placental barrier.
6. Draw the diagram of microanatomy of placenta.

Function of chorionic villi

_____

_____

_____

_____

Three points of identification

_____

_____

_____

_____

_____

_____

Date:

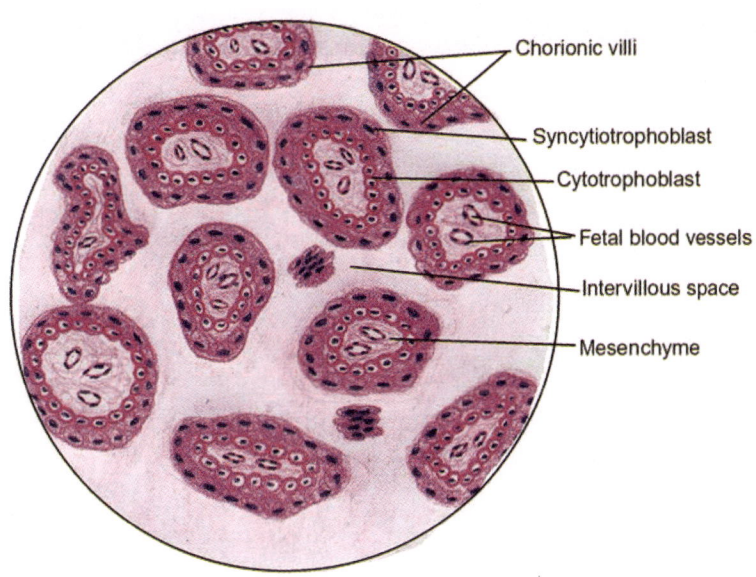

Chorionic villi

Syncytiotrophoblast

Cytotrophoblast

Fetal blood vessels

Intervillous space

Mesenchyme

Date:

UMBILICAL CORD

SPECIFIC LEARNING OBJECTIVES

At the end of the session the student should be able to:

1. Identify umbilical cord under the light microscope.
2. Identify two umbilical arteries and one umbilical vein.
3. Identify the Wharton's jelly which has fibroblasts, collagen fibres and ground substance which form the myxomatous tissue.
4. Identify the outer covering squamous epithelial cells of amnion.
5. Draw a diagram of microanatomy of umbilical cord.

Function of umbilical arteries and vein

_____

_____

_____

_____

Three points of identification

_____

_____

_____

_____

_____

_____

Date:

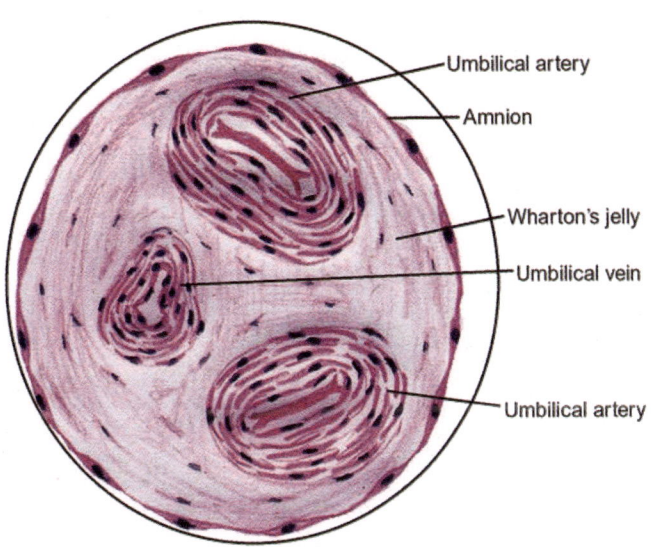

- Umbilical artery
- Amnion
- Wharton's jelly
- Umbilical vein
- Umbilical artery

Date:

SDL NOTES

Date:

CORPUS LUTEUM

Number	Competency	Domain	Level	Core (Y/N)	Teaching/learning method	Assessment method	Number required to certify
AN 52.3	Describe and identify the microanatomical features of cardioesophageal junction, corpus luteum	K/S	SH	Y	Lecture, practical	Written/skill assessment	

- Graffian follicle ruptures releasing the oocyte. The fluid in antrum is also released. The follicle collapses and later the granulosa cells and theca interna cells form corpus luteum.
- Granulosa cells and theca interna cells increase in size to form granulosa luteal cells and theca lutein cells respectively.
- If menstruation occurs then it forms corpus luteum of menstruation and if fertilisation occurs then it is known as corpus luteum of pregnancy.

Answer the Following

1. How is corpus luteum formed?

_____

_____

_____

_____

2. Which hormones are secreted by corpus luteum?

_____

_____

_____

_____

3. What happens to corpus luteum if fertilization fails to occur?

_____

_____

_____

_____

4. What happens to corpus luteum if fertilisation occurs?

_____

_____

_____

_____

Date:

SPECIFIC LEARNING OBJECTIVES

At the end of the session the student should be able to:

1. Identify corpus luteum under the light microscope.
2. Identify granulosa luteal cells.
3. Identify theca lutein cells.
4. Make a diagram of the microanatomy of corpus luteum.

Function of theca lutein cells

_____

_____

_____

_____

Three points of identification

_____

_____

_____

_____

_____

_____

Date:

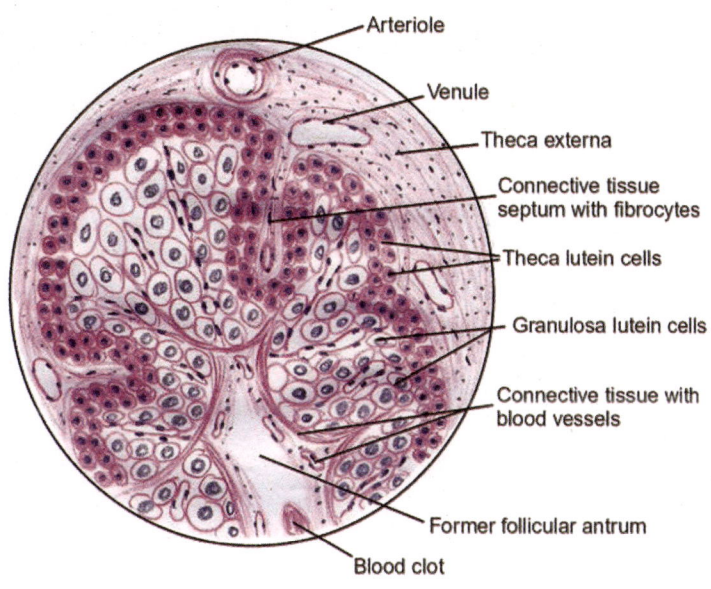

- Arteriole
- Venule
- Theca externa
- Connective tissue septum with fibrocytes
- Theca lutein cells
- Granulosa lutein cells
- Connective tissue with blood vessels
- Former follicular antrum
- Blood clot

Date:

BREAST

Number	Competency	Domain	Level	Core (Y/N)	Teaching/learning method	Assessment method	Number required to certify
AN 9.2	Breast: Describe the location, extent, deep relations, structure, age changes, blood supply, lymphatic drainage, microanatomy and applied anatomy of breast	K	KH	Y	Lecture, practical	Written viva voce	

- Mammary gland consists of 15–20 compound tubuloalveolar glands that form 15-20 lobes separated by connective tissue and fat. This interlobular connective tissue is more in resting mammary gland and reduces in mammary gland of pregnancy and lactation.
- Each gland opens at the nipple through lactiferous duct. These ducts have a dilatation beneath the nipple called lactiferous sinus.
- There are lobules in each lobe which have intralobular loose connective tissue which is devoid of fat. This connective tissue is also less in mammary gland of pregnancy and lactation.
- So there are intralobular, interlobular and lactiferous ducts.
- Lining epithelium rests on basement membrane. Between these two there are myoepithelial cells.

Date:

MAMMARY GLAND (RESTING)

SPECIFIC LEARNING OBJECTIVES

At the end of the session the student should be able to:

1. Identify resting mammary gland under the light microscope.
2. Identify intralobular and interlobular ducts of mammary glands.
3. Identify connective tissue between lobes.
4. Draw a diagram of microanatomy of resting mammary gland.

Function of intralobular and interlobular ducts of mammary glands

---

Three points of identification

Date:

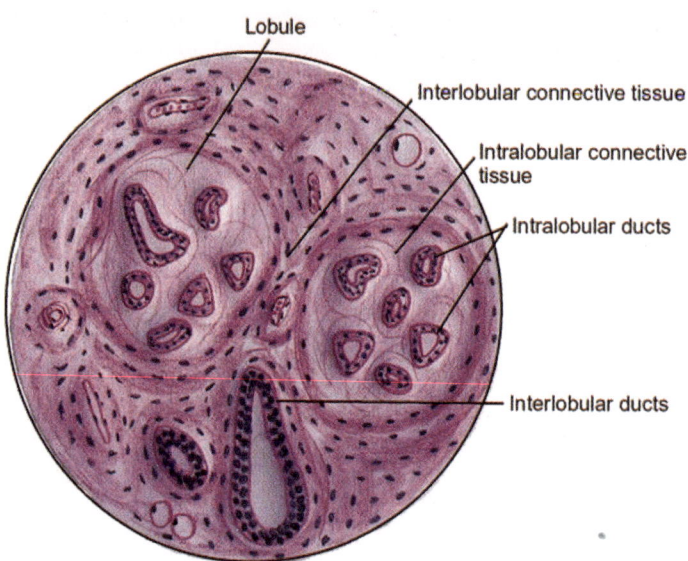

Lobule

Interlobular connective tissue

Intralobular connective tissue

Intralobular ducts

Interlobular ducts

Date:

MAMMARY GLAND OF PREGNANCY

SPECIFIC LEARNING OBJECTIVES

At the end of the session the student should be able to:

1. Identify mammary gland of pregnancy under the light microscope.
2. Identify presence of alveoli and interlobular and intralobular ducts.
3. Identify lesser connective tissue between lobes as compared from resting mammary gland.
4. Identify absence of fluid (milk) within alveoli.
5. Draw a diagram of microanatomy of mammary gland of pregnancy.

Function of myoepithelial cells in alveoli

_____

_____

_____

_____

Three points of identification

_____

_____

_____

_____

_____

_____

Date:

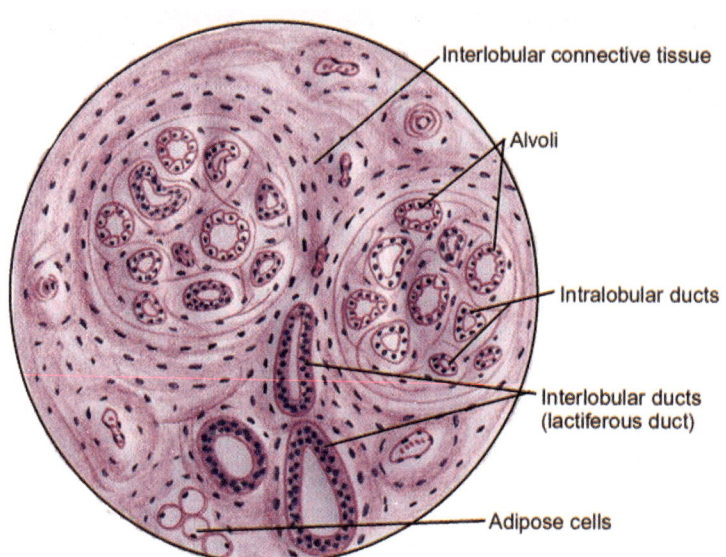

Interlobular connective tissue

Alvoli

Intralobular ducts

Interlobular ducts
(lactiferous duct)

Adipose cells

Date:

MAMMARY GLAND OF LACTATION

SPECIFIC LEARNING OBJECTIVES

At the end of the session the student should be able to:
1. Identify mammary gland of lactation under the light microscope.
2. Identify alveoli filled with fluid (milk).
3. Identify more alveoli and ducts than resting gland.
4. Identify less connective tissue than resting gland.
5. Draw a diagram of microanatomy of mammary gland of lactation.

Function of lactiferous ducts

_____

_____

_____

_____

Three points of identification

_____

_____

_____

_____

_____

_____

Date:

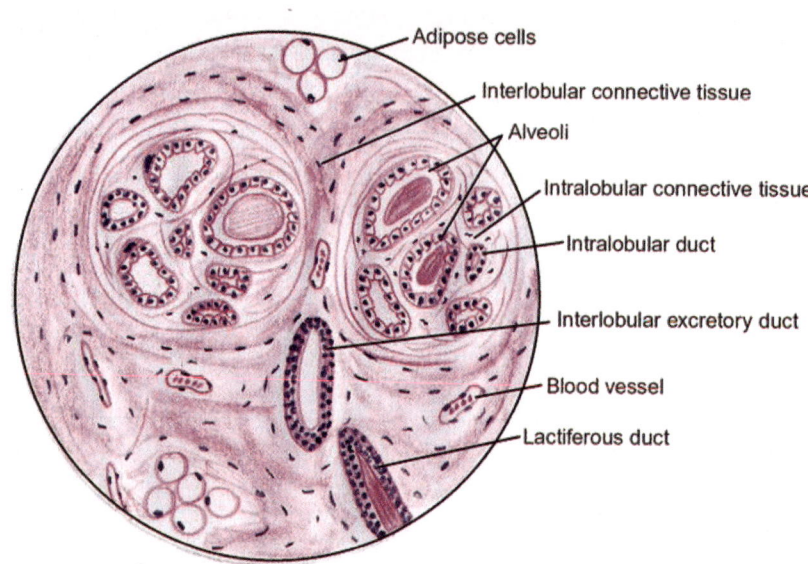

- Adipose cells
- Interlobular connective tissue
- Alveoli
- Intralobular connective tissue
- Intralobular duct
- Interlobular excretory duct
- Blood vessel
- Lactiferous duct

Date:

SDL NOTES

Date:

SDL NOTES

Date:

ENDOCRINE GLANDS

Number	Competency	Domain	Level	Core (Y/N)	Teaching/learning method	Assessment method	Number required to certify
AN 43.2	Identify, describe and draw the microanatomy of pituitary gland, thyroid, parathyroid gland, tongue, salivary glands, tonsil, epiglottis, cornea, retina	K/S	SH	Y	Lecture, practical	Written/skill assessment	

PITUITARY GLAND

- Pars anterior has cords of cells with fenestrated sinusoids between them. The cells are chromophil cells (acidophilic cells, basophilic cells) and chromophobe cells.
- Pars tuberalis has mostly undifferentiated cells.
- Pars intermedia has colloid filled vesicles which are remnants of Rathke's pouch.
- Pars posterior has unmyelinated nerve fibres of neurons of hypothalamus.
- Pituicytes are supporting cells in posterior pituitary.
- Axons terminals in posterior pituitary have secretory terminals called Herring bodies.

Date:

SPECIFIC LEARNING OBJECTIVES

At the end of the session the student should be able to:
1. Identify pituitary gland under the light microscope.
2. Identify pars anterior, pars intermedia, and pars posterior.
3. Identify chromophil and chromophobe cells.
4. Draw a diagram of microanatomy of pituitary gland.

Function of chromophil and chromophobe cells

_____

_____

_____

_____

Three points of identification

_____

_____

_____

_____

_____

_____

Date:

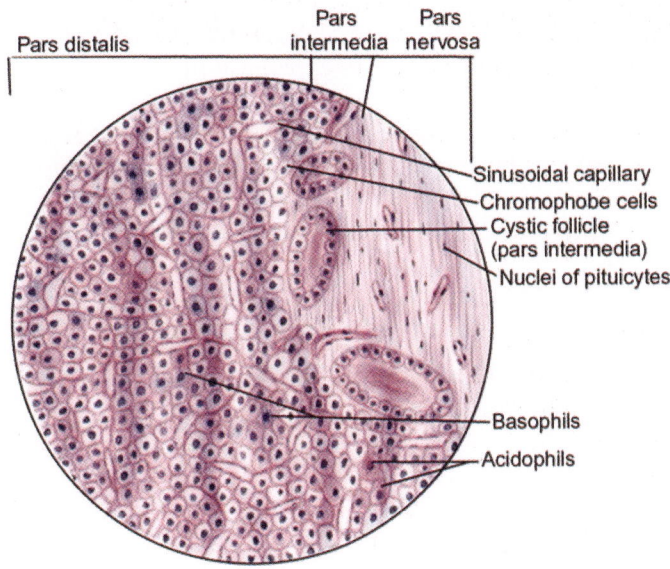

Pars distalis   Pars intermedia   Pars nervosa

Sinusoidal capillary
Chromophobe cells
Cystic follicle (pars intermedia)
Nuclei of pituicytes

Basophils

Acidophils

Date:

THYROID GLAND

- The thyroid gland is covered by a connective tissue capsule which sends septae within the gland carrying blood vessels and nerves.
- A section shows thyroid follicles filled with colloid which stains pink in H & E staining and is lined by simple cuboidal epithelium. The cells rest on a basement membrane. The surfaces of follicular cells towards the lumen have microvilli.
- Parafollicular/'C' cells are also present in clusters between the follicles. They stain pale as compared to the follicular cells.

SPECIFIC LEARNING OBJECTIVES

At the end of the session the student should be able to:

1. Identify thyroid gland under the light microscope.
2. Identify colloid filled thyroid follicles.
3. Identify simple cuboidal epithelium.
4. Identify parafollicular cells.
5. Draw a diagram of microanatomy of thyroid gland.

Function of thyroid follicles and parafollicular cells

_____

_____

_____

_____

Three points of identification

_____

_____

_____

_____

_____

_____

Date:

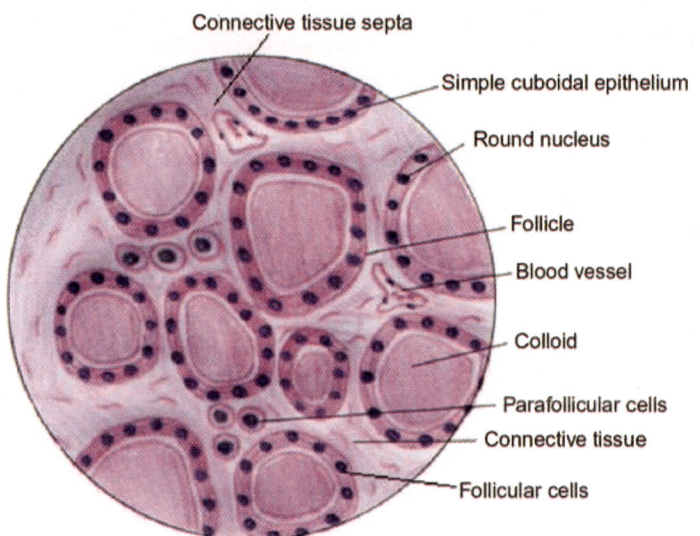

Connective tissue septa

Simple cuboidal epithelium

Round nucleus

Follicle

Blood vessel

Colloid

Parafollicular cells

Connective tissue

Follicular cells

Date:

PARATHYROID GLAND

- Two pairs of parathyroid glands are present on the posterior aspect of thyroid gland.
- Parathyroid gland has numerous principal cells/chief cells that are polygonal in shape. Nucleus is central in these cells.
- Oxyphil cells are also present. They are larger but lesser in number.

SPECIFIC LEARNING OBJECTIVES

At the end of the session the student should be able to:

1. Identify parathyroid gland under the light microscope.
2. Identify chief cell and oxyphil cells.
3. Draw a diagram of the microanatomy of parathyroid gland.

Function of chief and oxyphil cells of parathyroid gland

_____

_____

_____

_____

Three points of identification

_____

_____

_____

_____

_____

_____

Date:

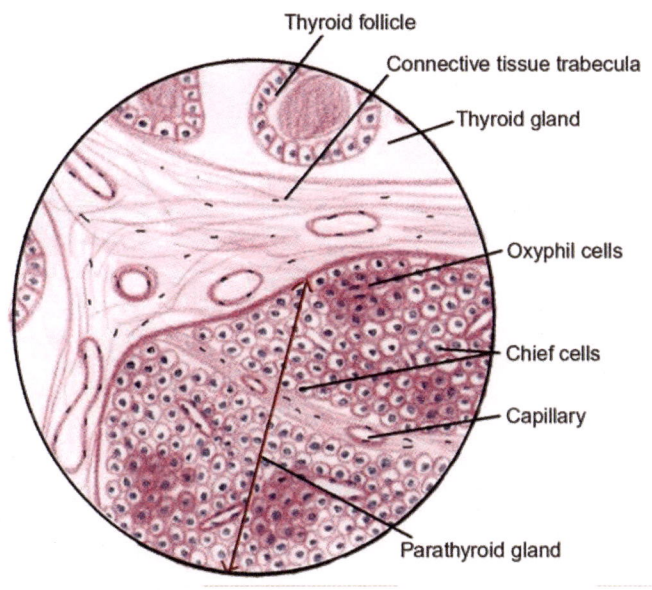

Thyroid follicle

Connective tissue trabecula

Thyroid gland

Oxyphil cells

Chief cells

Capillary

Parathyroid gland

Date:

SDL NOTES

Date:

PINEAL GLAND

Number	Competency	Domain	Level	Core (Y/N)	Teaching/learning method	Assessment method	Number required to certify
AN 43.3	Identify, describe and draw microanatomy of olfactory epithelium, eyelid, lip, sclera-corneal junction, optic nerve, cochlea-organ of Corti, pineal gland	K/S	SH	N	Lecture, practical	Written/skill assessment	

- A section shows calcified masses called corpora arenacea or brain sand. Corpora arenacea stains dark blue with H & E staining.
- The pineal gland is covered with piamater.
- 95% of the cells present in it are pinealocytes. They are polyhedral with large oval nucleus. Neuroglial cells, mainly astrocytes lie in between the pinealocytes.

SPECIFIC LEARNING OBJECTIVES

At the end of the session the student should be able to:
1. Identify pineal gland under the light microscope.
2. Identify corpora arenacea.
3. Identify pinealocytes and neuroglial cells.
4. Draw a diagram of microanatomy of pineal gland.

Function of pinealocytes

_____

_____

_____

_____

Three points of identification

_____

_____

_____

_____

_____

_____

Date:

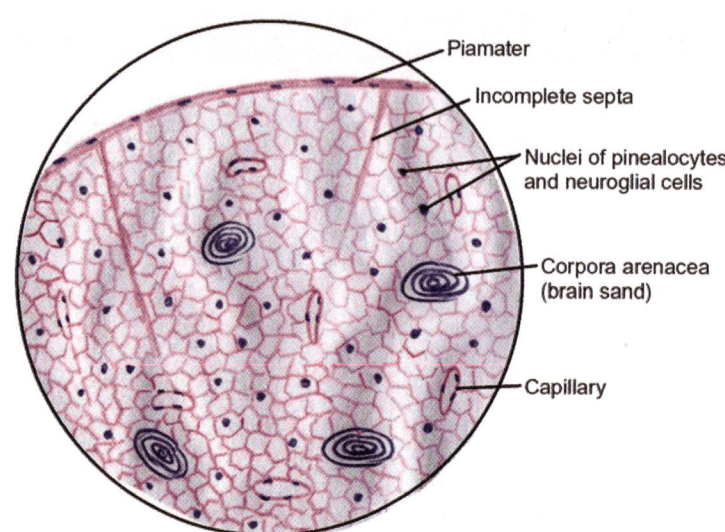

- Piamater
- Incomplete septa
- Nuclei of pinealocytes and neuroglial cells
- Corpora arenacea (brain sand)
- Capillary

Date:

SUPRARENAL GLAND

Number	Competency	Domain	Level	Core (Y/N)	Teaching/learning method	Assessment method	Number required to certify
AN 52.1	Describe and identify the microanatomical features of gastro-intestinal system: Oesophagus, fundus of stomach, pylorus of stomach, duodenum, jejunum, ileum, large intestine, appendix, liver gall bladder, pancreas and suprarenal gland	K/S	SH	Y	Lecture, practical	Written/skill assessment	

- Suprarenal gland has outer cortex (develops from coelomic epithelium, i.e. mesoderm) and inner medulla (develops from neural crest cells, i.e. ectoderm).
- Outermost covering capsule has capillaries.
- Cortex has three zones: outermost- zona glomerulosa, middle- zona fasciculata and innermost- zona reticularis. Capillaries are also present.
- Under the light microscope zona glomerulosa shows loops of basophilic columnar cells with dark spherical nuclei and sinusoids in between the cell groups. Mineralocorticoids are secreted by these cells.
- Zona fasciculata has vertical columns of cells which appear light basophilic stained due to large number of vacuoles. They are known as spongiocytes. They secrete glucorticoids. Vertical sinusoids also run along the columns of cells. Capillaries are also seen.
- Zona reticularis has a network of polygonal cells. They secrete sex steroid hormones. Capillaries can be seen in between.
- Medulla has two types of cells—chromaffin cells (phaeochromocytes) (more numerous) and ganglion cells. Medullary capillaries are also seen.
- Chromaffin cells are basophilic. The granules in the cytoplasm are precursors of epinephrine/adrenalin and noradrenaline.
- Ganglion cells are interspersed between the chromaffin cells. They are larger than chromaffin cells and have big nuclei with nucleoli.

Answer the Following

1. What are the three zones in cortex of suprarenal gland?

_____

_____

_____

2. What is the embryological origin of cortex and medulla of suprarenal gland? Correlate it with type of secretions.

_____

_____

_____

_____

_____

Date:

SPECIFIC LEARNING OBJECTIVES

At the end of the session the student should be able to:

1. Identify suprarenal gland under the light microscope.
2. Identify cortex and its three zones.
3. Identify medulla and its component cells.
4. Draw a diagram of microanatomy of suprarenal gland.

Function of three layers of cortex

_____

_____

_____

_____

Three points of identification

_____

_____

_____

_____

_____

_____

Date:

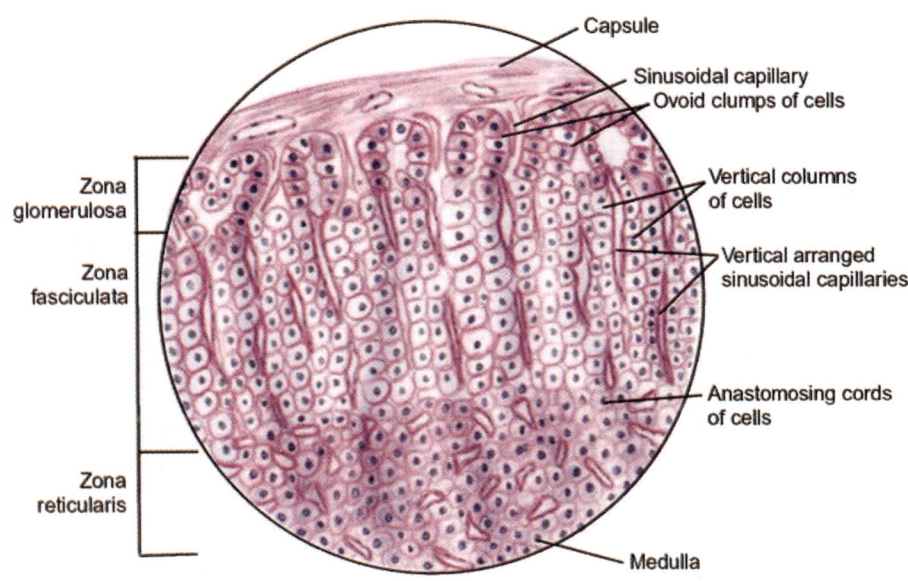

Capsule

Sinusoidal capillary

Ovoid clumps of cells

Zona glomerulosa

Vertical columns of cells

Zona fasciculata

Vertical arranged sinusoidal capillaries

Anastomosing cords of cells

Zona reticularis

Medulla

Date:

SDL NOTES

Date:

SDL NOTES

Date:

CENTRAL NERVOUS SYSTEM

Number	Competency	Domain	Level	Core (Y/N)	Teaching/learning method	Assessment method	Number required to certify
AN 64.1	Describe and identify the microanatomical features of spinal cord, cerebellum and cerebrum	K/S	SH	Y	Lecture, practical	Written/skill assessment	

SPINAL CORD

SPECIFIC LEARNING OBJECTIVES

At the end of the session the student should be able to:

1. Identify spinal cord under the light microscope.
2. Identify white matter and H-shaped grey matter.
3. Identify anterior horn cells.
4. Draw a diagram of microanatomy of spinal cord.

Function of anterior horn cells

_____

_____

_____

_____

Three points of identification

_____

_____

_____

_____

_____

_____

Date:

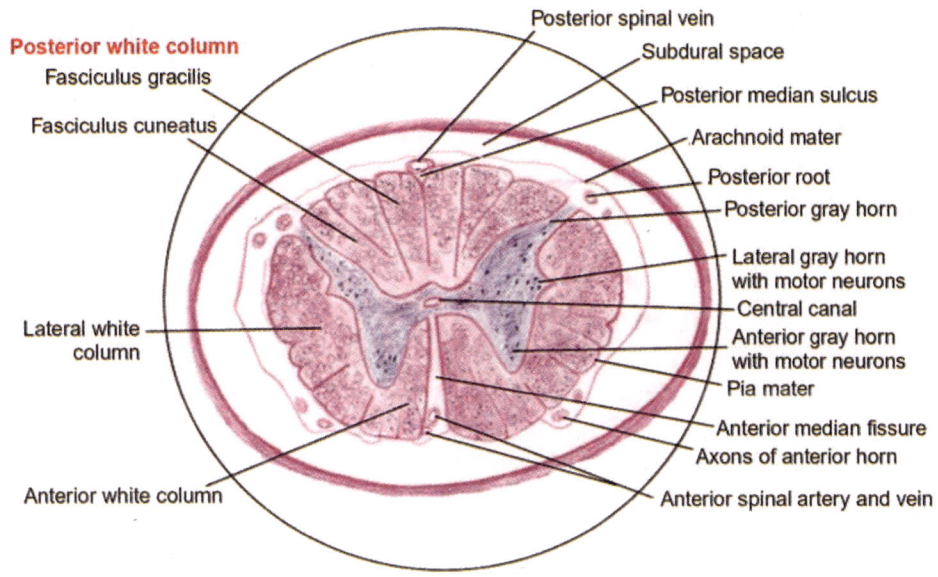

Posterior white column
Fasciculus gracilis
Fasciculus cuneatus
Lateral white column
Anterior white column

Posterior spinal vein
Subdural space
Posterior median sulcus
Arachnoid mater
Posterior root
Posterior gray horn
Lateral gray horn with motor neurons
Central canal
Anterior gray horn with motor neurons
Pia mater
Anterior median fissure
Axons of anterior horn
Anterior spinal artery and vein

Date:

SDL NOTES

Date:

CEREBRUM

SPECIFIC LEARNING OBJECTIVES

At the end of the session the student should be able to:
1. Identify cerebrum under the light microscope.
2. Identify small, medium and large pyramidal cells.
3. Identify the six layers of cerebral cortex.
4. Draw a diagram of microanatomy of cerebrum.

Function of pyramidal cells

_____

_____

_____

_____

Three points of identification

_____

_____

_____

_____

_____

_____

Date:

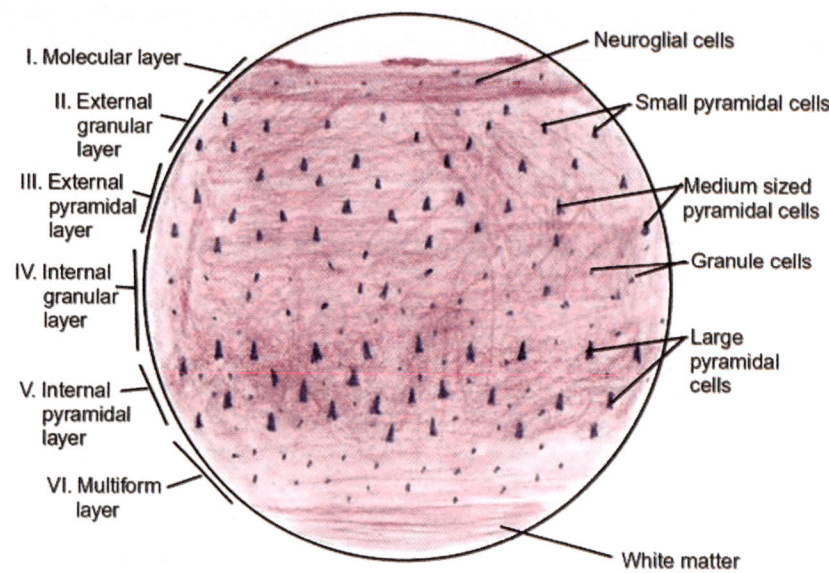

I. Molecular layer

II. External granular layer

III. External pyramidal layer

IV. Internal granular layer

V. Internal pyramidal layer

VI. Multiform layer

Neuroglial cells

Small pyramidal cells

Medium sized pyramidal cells

Granule cells

Large pyramidal cells

White matter

Date:

CEREBELLUM

SPECIFIC LEARNING OBJECTIVES

At the end of the session the student should be able to:

1. Identify cerebellum under the light microscope.
2. Identify folia of cerebellum.
3. Identify grey matter and white matter of cerebellum.
4. Identify the three layers of grey matter.
5. Identify Purkinje cells of middle layer.
6. Draw a labelled diagram of microstructure of cerebellum.

Function of Purkinje cells

_____

_____

_____

_____

Three points of identification

_____

_____

_____

_____

_____

_____

Date:

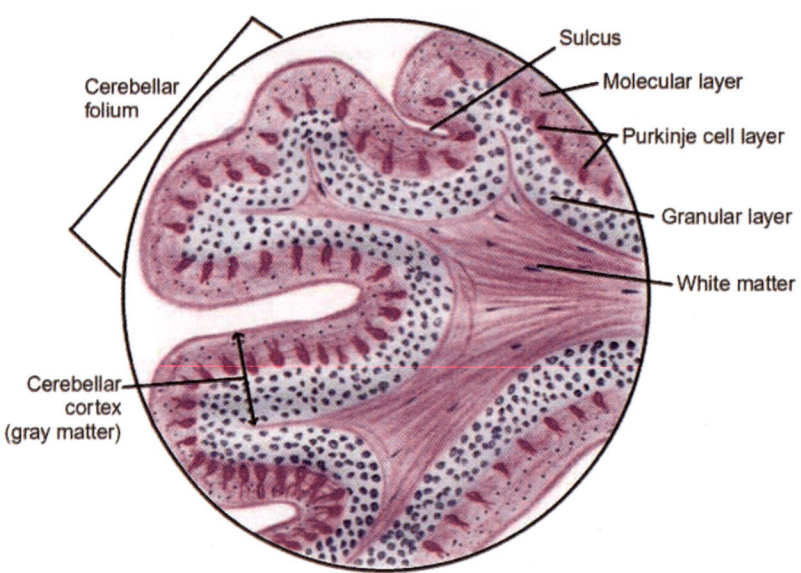

Cerebellar folium

Sulcus

Molecular layer

Purkinje cell layer

Granular layer

White matter

Cerebellar cortex (gray matter)

Date:

SDL NOTES

Date:

SDL NOTES

Date:

SPECIAL SENSES

Number	Competency	Domain	Level	Core (Y/N)	Teaching/learning method	Assessment method	Number required to certify
AN 43.2	Identify, describe and draw the microanatomy of pituitary gland, thyroid, parathyroid gland, tongue, salivary glands, tonsil, epiglottis, cornea, retina	K/S	SH	Y	Lecture, practical	Written/skill assessment	
AN 43.3	Identify, describe and draw microanatomy of olfactory epithelium, eyelid, lip, sclero-corneal junction, optic nerve, cochlea- organ of corti, pineal gland	K/S	SH	N	Lecture, practical	Written/skill assessment	

CORNEA

Cornea has five layers:
1. **Corneal epithelium** (Stratified squamous non-keratinised). Cells near the base are columnar, middle ones polygonal and superficial squamous.
2. **Bowman's membrane (anterior limiting membrane):** Epithelium rests on this membrane.
3. **Corneal stroma/substantia propria:** Made up of type 1 collagen fibres present in ground substance. Both have the same refractive index which makes the cornea transparent. Fibroblasts in substantia propria are called keratocytes.
4. **Descemet's membrane:** It is a thin homogenous layer (appears unstained in H & E) also known as posterior limiting membrane (anterior limiting membrane being Bowman's membrane). It continues with fibres in irido-corneal angle.
5. **Endothelium:** It may be squamous or cuboidal epithelium.

Answer the Following

Why is cornea transparent?

_____

_____

_____

_____

_____

_____

_____

_____

Date:

SPECIFIC LEARNING OBJECTIVES

At the end of the session the student should be able to:

1. Identify cornea under the light microscope.
2. Identify the five layers of cornea.
3. Draw a diagram of the microanatomy of cornea.

Correlate microanatomical structure of cornea with its function

_____

_____

_____

_____

Three points of identification

_____

_____

_____

_____

_____

_____

Date:

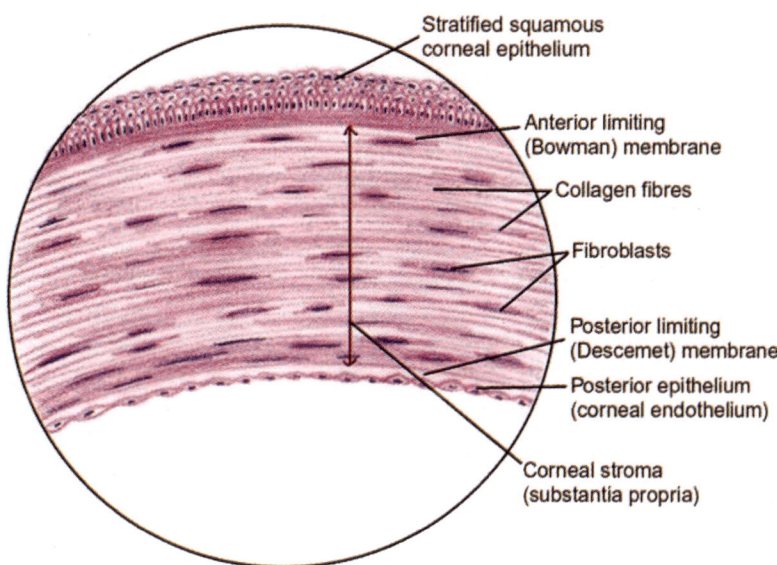

Stratified squamous
corneal epithelium

Anterior limiting
(Bowman) membrane

Collagen fibres

Fibroblasts

Posterior limiting
(Descemet) membrane

Posterior epithelium
(corneal endothelium)

Corneal stroma
(substantia propria)

Date:

SCLERO-CORNEAL JUNCTION

- The sclera (outermost layer of eyeball) consists of bundles of fibrous tissue running parallel to the surface. It has fibroblasts and few elastic fibres. It is opaque.
- Cornea has the five layers described earlier. It is transparent.
- The marginal zone is called limbus. The transition of epithelium to that of conjunctiva is gradual and not well-demarcated.
- Bowman's membrane of cornea ends here and loose connective tissue beneath the epithelium begins. Bowman's membrane becomes continuous with lamina propria of conjunctiva and Tenon's capsule.
- There is a trabecular meshwork just near the periphery of Descemet's membrane. Spaces between this meshwork are known as spaces of Fontana.
- Descemet's membrane tapers at the anterior limbal boundary and posterior portion becomes interlaced with trabecular meshwork. It becomes Schwalbe's line.
- Corneal endothelium continues in the anterior chamber angle as endothelial covering of the trabecular meshwork.
- Conjunctival stroma has no counterpart in the cornea.
- Just behind the sclero-corneal junction there is a circular channel called canal of Schlemm in the sclera.
- Medial to the canal of Schlemm there is a triangular projection of sclera tissue called sclera spur.

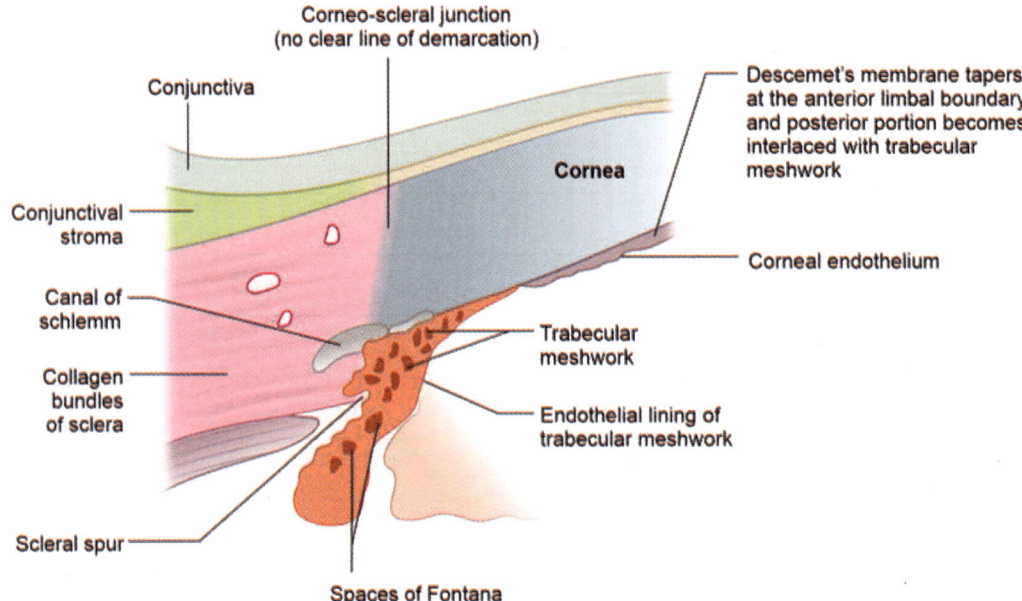

Date:

SPECIFIC LEARNING OBJECTIVES

At the end of the session the student should be able to:
1. Identify the sclero-corneal junction under the light microscope.
2. Identify the trabecular meshwork.
3. Identify the scleral spur.
4. Identify the canal of Schlemm.
5. Draw a diagram of the microanatomy of sclero-corneal junction.

Function of canal of Schlemm

_____

_____

_____

_____

Three points of identification

_____

_____

_____

_____

_____

_____

Date:

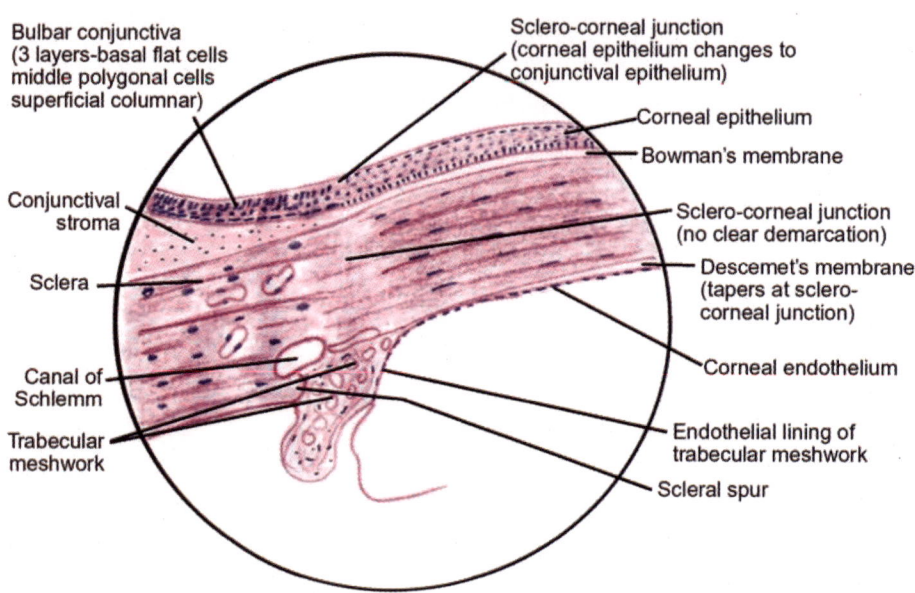

Bulbar conjunctiva
(3 layers-basal flat cells
middle polygonal cells
superficial columnar)

Conjunctival
stroma

Sclera

Canal of
Schlemm

Trabecular
meshwork

Sclero-corneal junction
(corneal epithelium changes to
conjunctival epithelium)

Corneal epithelium

Bowman's membrane

Sclero-corneal junction
(no clear demarcation)

Descemet's membrane
(tapers at sclero-
corneal junction)

Corneal endothelium

Endothelial lining of
trabecular meshwork

Scleral spur

Date:

RETINA

Just like the rest of the organs, we must know the various cells and fibres arranged in the retina to understand its microscopic structure. They are as shown in the diagram below:

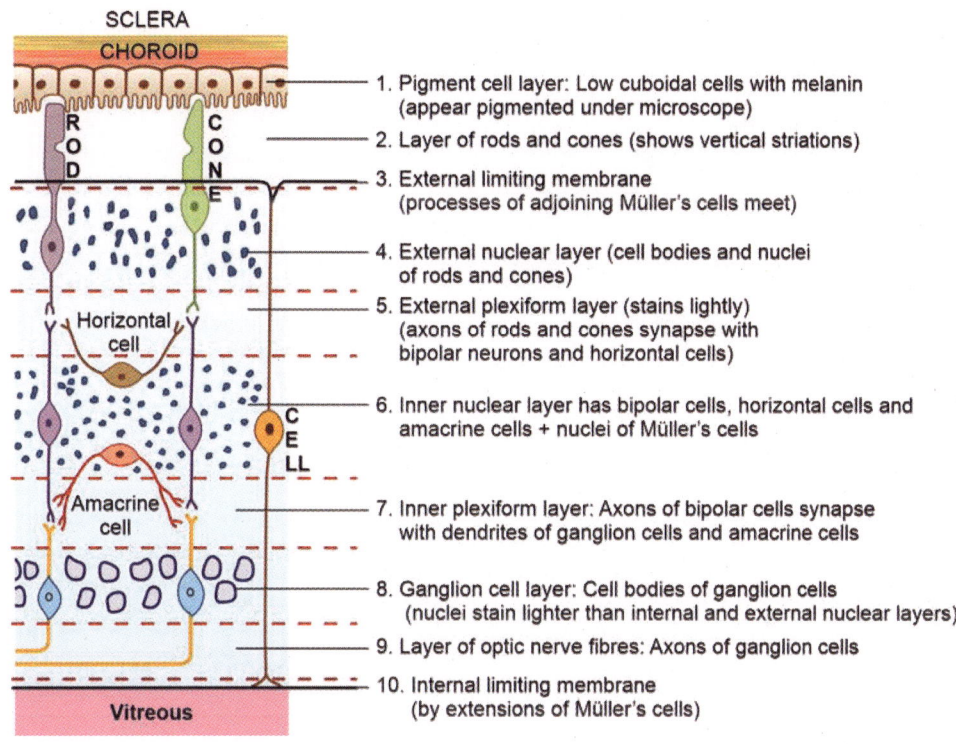

1. Pigment cell layer: Low cuboidal cells with melanin (appear pigmented under microscope)
2. Layer of rods and cones (shows vertical striations)
3. External limiting membrane (processes of adjoining Müller's cells meet)
4. External nuclear layer (cell bodies and nuclei of rods and cones)
5. External plexiform layer (stains lightly) (axons of rods and cones synapse with bipolar neurons and horizontal cells)
6. Inner nuclear layer has bipolar cells, horizontal cells and amacrine cells + nuclei of Müller's cells
7. Inner plexiform layer: Axons of bipolar cells synapse with dendrites of ganglion cells and amacrine cells
8. Ganglion cell layer: Cell bodies of ganglion cells (nuclei stain lighter than internal and external nuclear layers)
9. Layer of optic nerve fibres: Axons of ganglion cells
10. Internal limiting membrane (by extensions of Müller's cells)

Date:

SPECIFIC LEARNING OBJECTIVES

At the end of the session the student should be able to:

1. Identify retina under the light microscope.
2. Identify the layers of retina-pigment layer, layer of rods and cones, external nuclear layer, external plexiform layer, inner nuclear layer, internal plexiform layer, layer of ganglion cells, layer of optic nerve fibres.
3. Draw a diagram of microanatomy of retina.

Function of pigment layer of retina

_____

_____

_____

_____

Three points of identification

_____

_____

_____

_____

_____

_____

Date:

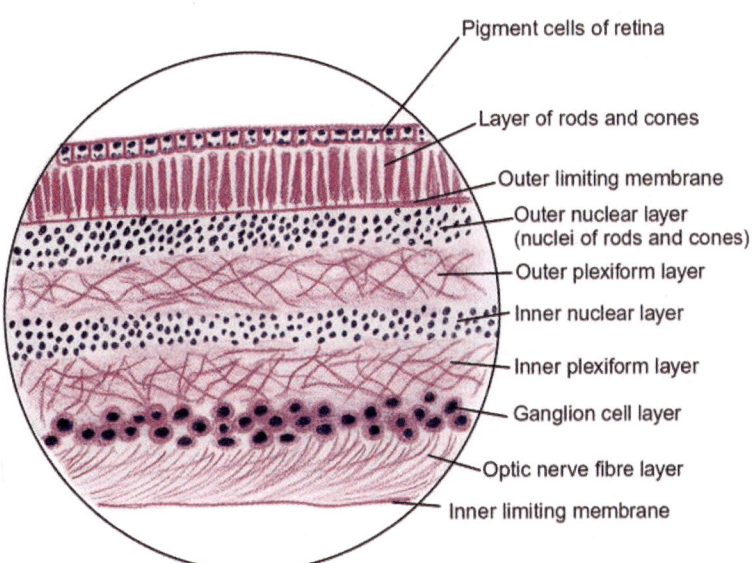

Pigment cells of retina

Layer of rods and cones

Outer limiting membrane

Outer nuclear layer
(nuclei of rods and cones)

Outer plexiform layer

Inner nuclear layer

Inner plexiform layer

Ganglion cell layer

Optic nerve fibre layer

Inner limiting membrane

Date:

SDL NOTES

OPTIC NERVE

Number	Competency	Domain	Level	Core (Y/N)	Teaching/learning method	Assessment method	Number required to certify
AN 43.2	Identify, describe and draw microanatomy of olfactory epithelium, eyelid, lip, sclero-corneal junction, optic nerve, cochlea-organ of Corti, pineal gland	K/S	SH	N	Lecture, practical	Written/skill assessment	

SPECIFIC LEARNING OBJECTIVES

At the end of the session the student should be able to:
1. Identify optic nerve under the light microscope.
2. Identify bundles of axons of ganglion cells.
3. Identify central retinal vein and central retinal artery.
4. Draw a diagram of microanatomy of optic nerve.

Differentiate between peripheral and optic nerve

_____

_____

_____

_____

Three points of identification

_____

_____

_____

_____

_____

_____

Date:

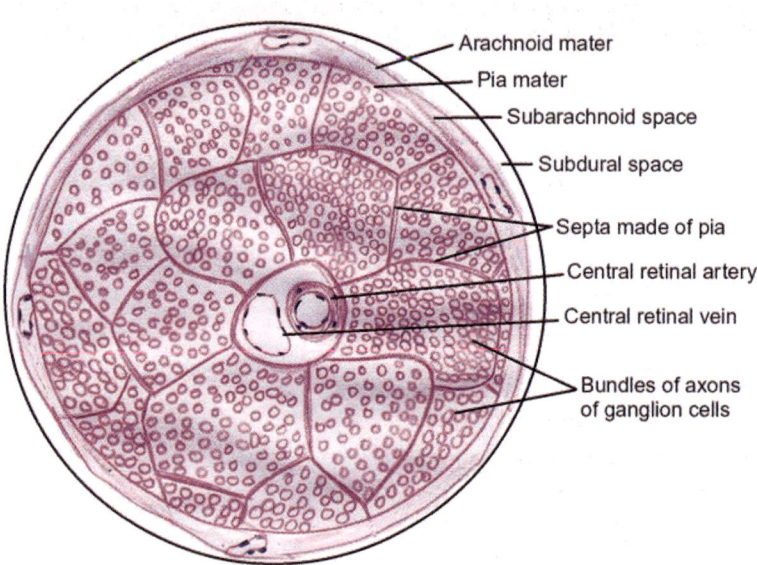

- Arachnoid mater
- Pia mater
- Subarachnoid space
- Subdural space
- Septa made of pia
- Central retinal artery
- Central retinal vein
- Bundles of axons of ganglion cells

Date:

EYELID

- Eyelid has two surfaces—anterior surface is a layer of thin skin and posterior layer is of palpebral conjunctiva (striated columnar epithelium).
- Connective tissue beneath thin skin is devoid of fat.
- Deep to skin there is skeletal muscle (orbicularis oculi).
- Then there is tarsal plate which is dense fibrous tissue.
- Deep to tarsal plate there are tarsal glands (Meibomian glands). The ducts of each of these glands open at the free margin of eyelid. They are modified sebaceous glands. Each acinus of the gland contains a large number of large, pale-staining, polygonal cells, all of which are surrounded by a single layer of smaller cells called basal cells. The cytoplasm of these cells stain poorly due to accumulation of sebum which does not take H & E stain. Basal cells do not contain sebum, so they take up the stain.
- Ciliary glands (glands of Moll) are present near the free edge of eyelid. They are modified sweat glands.
- Glands of Zeis are sebaceous glands opening in the hair follicles of eyelids.
- Glands of Wolfring (accessory lacrimal glands) are present above the tarsal plate.

Think and Answer

1. What are the layers of thin skin?

_____

_____

_____

_____

2. What is the function of tarsal plate?

_____

_____

_____

_____

3. What is a stye?

_____

_____

_____

_____

4. What is a chalazion?

_____

_____

_____

_____

_____

Date:

SPECIFIC LEARNING OBJECTIVES

At the end of the session the student should be able to:

1. Identify eyelid under the light microscope.
2. Identify palpebral conjunctiva and thin skin.
3. Identify tarsal plate and tarsal gland.
4. Identify skeletal muscle.
5. Identify eyelash and its hair follicle.
6. Draw a diagram of microanatomy of eyelid.

Function of tarsal plate

_____

_____

_____

Three points of identification

_____

_____

_____

_____

_____

_____

Date:

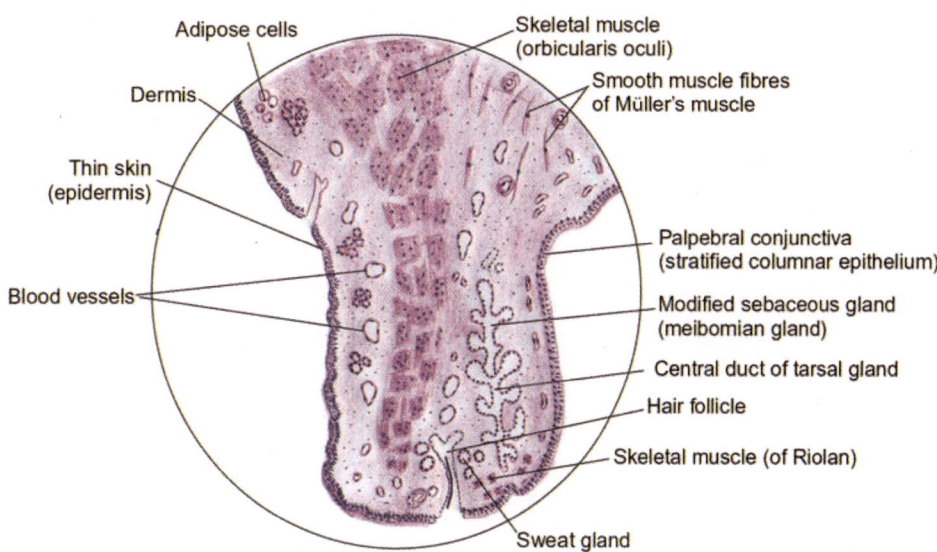

Adipose cells

Dermis

Thin skin
(epidermis)

Blood vessels

Skeletal muscle
(orbicularis oculi)

Smooth muscle fibres
of Müller's muscle

Palpebral conjunctiva
(stratified columnar epithelium)

Modified sebaceous gland
(meibomian gland)

Central duct of tarsal gland

Hair follicle

Skeletal muscle (of Riolan)

Sweat gland

Date:

SDL NOTES

Date:

LIP

SPECIFIC LEARNING OBJECTIVES

At the end of the session the student should be able to:

1. Identify lip under the light microscope.
2. Identify skin, vermillion border and oral mucosa.
3. Identify hair follicles, sebaceous glands and sweat glands in skin.
4. Identify serous and mucous glands in submucosa (under mucosa on the inner side).
5. Identify orbicularis oris (skeletal muscle).
6. Draw a diagram of microanatomy of lip.

Function of oral mucosa

_____

_____

_____

_____

Three points of identification

_____

_____

_____

_____

_____

_____

Date:

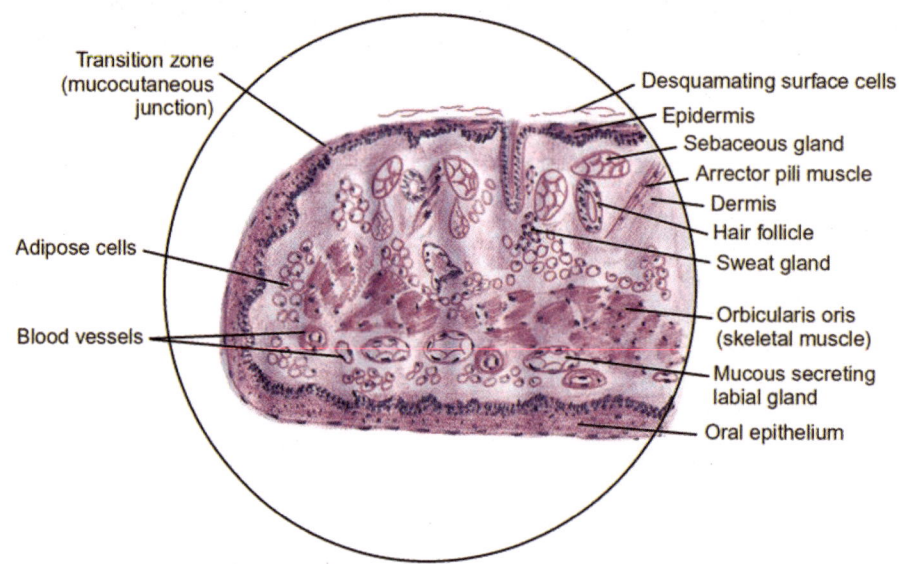

- Transition zone (mucocutaneous junction)
- Desquamating surface cells
- Epidermis
- Sebaceous gland
- Arrector pili muscle
- Dermis
- Hair follicle
- Sweat gland
- Adipose cells
- Orbicularis oris (skeletal muscle)
- Blood vessels
- Mucous secreting labial gland
- Oral epithelium

Date:

COCHLEA AND ORGAN OF CORTI

What is bony labyrinth and membranous labyrinth?

- Labyrinth literally means a complex irregular network of passages. Bony labyrinth is a hollow meshwork of cavities in the temporal bone in which lies the inner ear (vestibule, semicircular canals and cochlea).
- Membranous labyrinth is a collection of tubes (i.e. soft tissue) which are filled with fluid. They contain receptors for the senses of balance and hearing.

What is cochlea?

It is a spiral tube of the inner ear cavity containing organ of Corti which produces nerve impulses in response to sound vibrations. It appears like a shell of a snail. The tube spirals 2 3/4th times around a bony projection called modiolus.

How is cochlea divided?

A shelf-like projection from the modiolus divides the cochlea incompletely into one tube above called scala vestibuli and one tube below called scala tympani. Both these communicate at the apex through helicotrema. In the middle is the organ of Corti which has another scala called scala media.

What is the organ of Corti and where is it found?

Organ of Corti is the receptor organ for hearing found in the cochlea between scala vestibuli and scala tympani.

What cells are found in the organ of Corti?

Single row of inner hair cells, 3 rows of outer hair cells, pillar cells, Deiter's cells (also known as phalangeal cells), Hensen's cells, supporting cells.

What are the other structures found in the organ of Corti and cochlear duct?

- Reticular membrane—formed by apices of outer hair cells and phalangeal cells.
- Basilar membrane—extends from the tip of spiral lamina of modiolus to the outer wall of cochlea. It separates cochlear duct from scala tympani.
- Tectorial membrane—it is gelatinous and produced by columnar cells on top of spiral limbus just medial to the organ of Corti.
- Reissner's membrane (vestibular membrane)—separates cochlear duct from scala vestibuli.

Date:

SPECIFIC LEARNING OBJECTIVES

At the end of the student should be able to:

1. Identify cochlea and organ of Corti under the light microscope.
2. Identify scala vestibuli, scala tympani and scala media.
3. Identify Reissner's membrane, tectorial membrane, basilar membrane and reticular membrane.
4. Identify inner and outer hair cells and tunnel of Corti.
5. Identify stria vascularis and limbus.
6. Draw a diagram of microanatomy of cochlea and organ of Corti.

Function of inner and outer hair cells of organ of Corti

_____

_____

_____

_____

Three points of identification

_____

_____

_____

_____

_____

_____

Date:

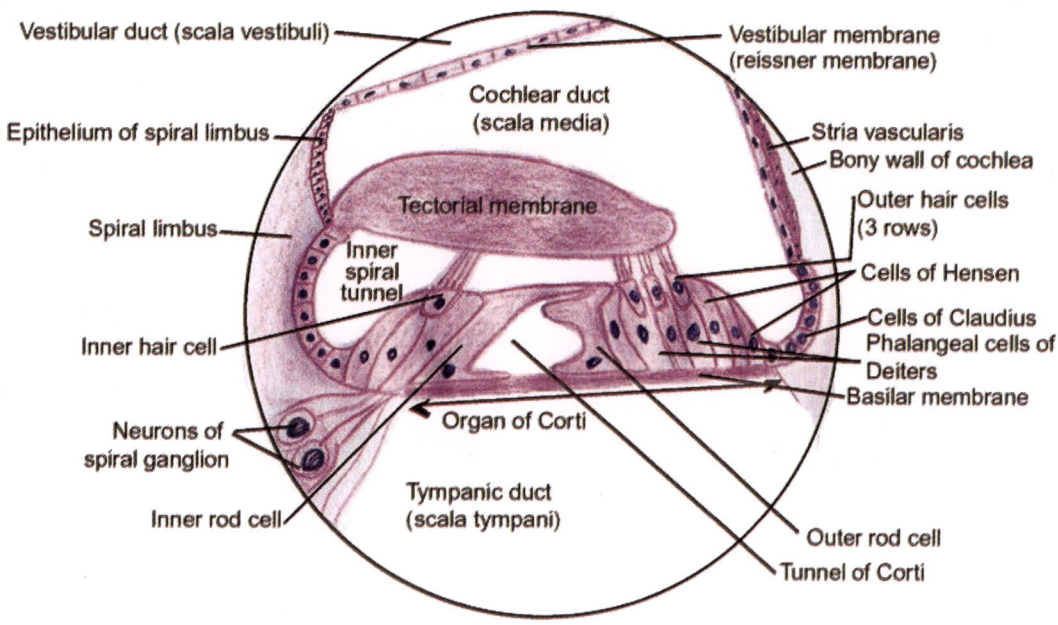

Vestibular duct (scala vestibuli)

Epithelium of spiral limbus

Spiral limbus

Inner hair cell

Neurons of spiral ganglion

Inner rod cell

Cochlear duct (scala media)

Tectorial membrane

Inner spiral tunnel

Organ of Corti

Tympanic duct (scala tympani)

Vestibular membrane (reissner membrane)

Stria vascularis
Bony wall of cochlea

Outer hair cells (3 rows)

Cells of Hensen

Cells of Claudius
Phalangeal cells of Deiters

Basilar membrane

Outer rod cell
Tunnel of Corti

Date:

SDL NOTES

Date:

SDL NOTES

ABBREVIATIONS

1. SLO: Specific learning objectives
2. H & E: Haematoxylin and eosin
3. LS: Longitudinal section
4. ECM: Extracellular matrix
5. BM: Bone marrow
6. LN: Lymph node
7. WBC: White blood cells
8. RBCs: Red blood cells
9. SDL: Self-directed learning
10. RER: Rough endoplasmic reticulum
11. SER: Smooth endoplasmic reticulum

Characteristics of Haematoxylin and Eosin Staining in Various Tissues and Different Parts of Cells

Basophilic	Violet (Blue)
Acidophilic	Lilac (Pink)
Cell membrane	Lilac (Pink)
Nucleus	Violet (Blue)
Cytoplasm	Lilac (Pink)
Nucleoplasm	Violet (Blue)
Nucleoli	Violet (Blue)
Basement membrane	Lilac (Pink)
Elastic fibres	Lilac (Pink)
Collagen fibres	Lilac (Pink)
Reticular fibres	Not stained by H & E
Elastic fibres of elastic cartilage	Lilac (Pink)
Hyaline cartilage	Homogenous
Mucous	Not stained by H & E
Serous inclusions	Violet (Blue)
Goblet cells	Not stained by H & E
Muscle fibres	Lilac (Pink) (except their nucleus)
Bone matrix	Lilac (Pink)
Nerve fibre	Lilac (Pink)
Lacunae in cartilage	Outline is Violet
Lacunae in bones	Outline is Violet
Microvilli	Lilac (Pink) – deep staining
Keratin	Lilac (Pink)
Cilia	Lilac (Pink)
Stereocilia	Lilac
Striated border	Dark pink (lilac)
Corpora amylacea	Eosinophilic (pink)
Lipid	No staining by H & E
Corpora arenacea	Basophilic (dark blue)

Date:

FEEDBACK FORM

1. Suggestions for improvement of diagrams

_____
_____
_____
_____
_____
_____
_____

2. Suggestions for improvement of content

_____
_____
_____
_____
_____
_____
_____
_____
_____

3. Any other suggestion

_____
_____
_____
_____
_____
_____
_____
_____
_____

Note: Suggestion may be mailed at *drsharmah@gmail.com* or messaged on contact number 9799970949.